I0788004

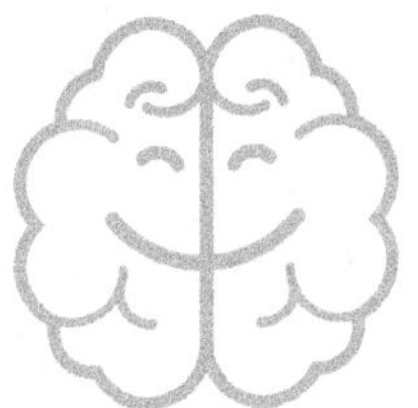

A HEAD ABOVE

A Simple Guide to Peak Mental Performance

ISBN   978-1-97413-706-0

MANSAL DENTON

A HEAD ABOVE

A SIMPLE GUIDE TO PEAK MENTAL PERFORMANCE

CONTENTS

INTRODUCTION

"Coffee, the sober drink, the mighty nourishment of the brain, which unlike other spirits, heightens purity and lucidity; coffee, which clears the clouds of the imagination and their gloomy weight; which illuminates the reality of things suddenly with the flash of truth."
—JULES MICHELET[1]

Prior to the mid-17th century, most Europeans drank wine, brandy, and beer for reasons far beyond mere social lubrication. Alcohol was safer to drink than water, so, in the name of health and well-being, they consumed glasses in the morning, afternoon, and evening.

The Europeans took this habit with them on colonial voyages. On the Mayflower, the English ship bringing the first Pilgrims to America, one William Wood observed: "It is thought that there can be no better water in the world, yet dare I not prefer it before good beer."[2]

---

1   Standage, Tom. *A History of the World in 6 Glasses*. London: Atlantic Books, 2007. P. 133.

2   Ibid., 114

Consuming alcohol may have been safer than water, but it left European intellectuals in a constant state of mild inebriation. A 1674 poem published by an anonymous author denounced wine as a "sweet Poison of the Treacherous Grape," which drowns "our very Reason and our Souls."[3] If there was one thing holding the thinkers of the day back, it was the constant alcoholic haze.

From Africa came the antidote. Europeans imported coffee, which altered the course of human history forever.

The scientists were the first to adopt coffee instead of alcohol. The first coffeehouse to open in Britain was in the university town of Oxford, where Francis Bacon, Isaac Newton, and others frequented. As the trend took hold, intellectuals, scientists, and merchants stopped drinking alcohol and started consuming caffeine-infused coffee. It's no surprise, then, that the spread of coffee mirrored the Age of Reason, the Scientific Revolution, and the Enlightenment.

The new ideas that sprang forward were giant leaps for mankind. We went from blindly believing ancient texts from religions and Greek philosophers to judging the world around us based on scientific reason and measurement.

The scientific discoveries laid the foundation for modern, technological growth. The same philosophies laid the groundwork for political reforms and freedoms, which many westerners enjoy today. It goes to show what can be achieved with a little cognitive enhancement.

----

3   Ibid., 135.

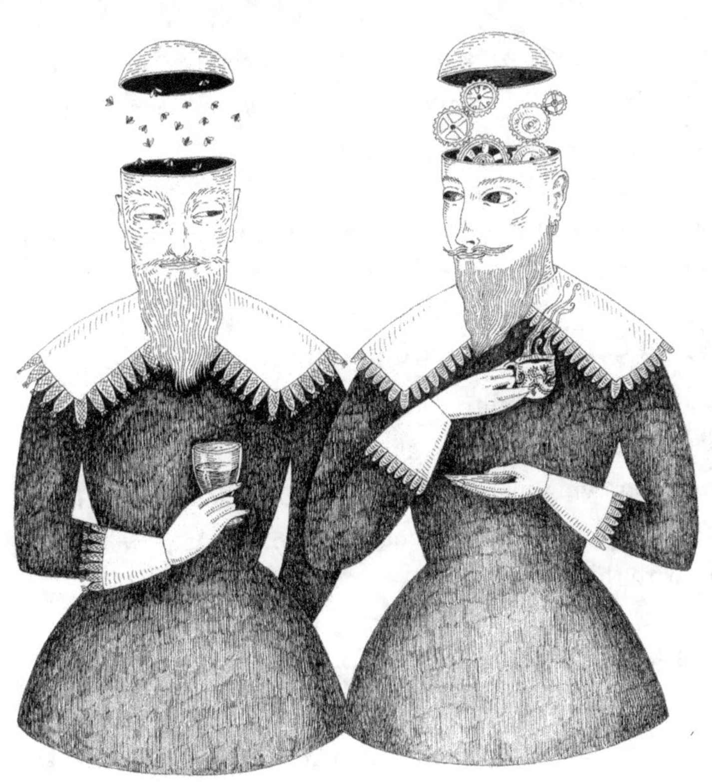

The same can be said of nootropics today. As philosopher and Oxford researcher Nick Bostrom suggests: "...if the ten million scientists in the world all benefited from the drug, the inventor would increase the rate of scientific progress by roughly the same amount as adding one hundred-thousand new scientists."[4]

Coffee alone did not create these paradigm shifts in human history, just as nootropics will not solve all of our greatest challenges.

---

4   Nick Bostrom, "Three Ways to Advance Science" for *Nature* podcast, Jan 2008.

But there is no denying the influence. When the brightest minds of the day trade mild inebriation for focus and mental clarity, we can far easier solve humanity's problems.

History shows, incremental and even 1% changes in human cognitive performance can go a long way.

Playing Catch Up with Cognition

A 1% change in cognitive performance might help society, but it doesn't sound like an attractive improvement for me. When I think about improving mental performance, I'm looking for far bigger numbers than a single percent—and, fortunately, this is still possible with the brain.

Cognitive enhancements can range anywhere from 8.6%, as is the case with the nootropic called piracetam (memory formation),[5] to 35% in a root nootropic called Rhodiola Rosea (anti-fatigue),[6] and even higher.

The reason we can achieve so much higher returns on our brain is that cognitive performance hasn't been a focus; until recently, cognitive enhancement and nootropics have been a relatively fringe phenomenon. Techniques to optimize mental performance are lagging compared to elite physical athletes and training programs. The attention, research, money, and, therefore, the advancements have been concentrated on the physical performance space.

---

5 Dimond SJ. "Increase in the power of human memory in normal man through the use of drugs." *Psychopharmacology*. Sep 29,1976.

6 Darbinyan V. "Clinical trial of Rhodiola rosea L. extract SHR-5 in the treatment of mild to moderate depression." *Nord J Psychiatry*. 2007.

Few people have tried or even heard of nootropics outside of sub-communities of Silicon Valley, Wall Street, or biohackers, whereas nearly every athlete supplements their diet with protein powders and pre-workouts.

The Olympics provide a perfect example of this disparity. The last two Olympic games[7] saw fifty-nine separate world records broken. These records were broken not because we give birth to genetically superior mutant babies, but instead because our training methods have gotten better.

With a better understanding of the body, recovery, and perfor-mance, the world's best athletes continue to excel.

Winning gold medals is great, but this is a lopsided distribution of our optimization efforts. We aren't prioritizing the right things. Consider that 40% of the western world's workforce is consid-ered "knowledge workers" (doctors, bankers, entrepreneurs, and just about anyone sitting inside at a desk). They all rely primarily on their mental performance for their livelihood. These are the people who create the technologies that solve global energy short-ages, cure life-threatening diseases, and put human colonies into space.

If society spends resources on optimizing mental vs. physical performance, we can solve great challenges. Individuals will be far more intelligent, focused, creative, and successful than their apathetic peers. The good news is that there is no need to wait.

---

7   2012 and 2016

We already have everything we need to get started at our disposal. Laying the foundation for enhanced cognition (and experiencing its benefits) can be done anywhere, by anyone, at any stage of life.

Why Cognitive Enhancement and Why Now?

Awaiting the daily mail is one of the few moments of excitement inside prison walls. Days usually follow the whims of prison guards, and there is little to look forward to. Even the television shows are reruns, making mailtime one of the few breaks from monotony.

Excitement may have accompanied mail time, but it rarely yielded any fruit. We all wanted a letter, though few people received one. Because I had no freedom or regular communication with the outside world, the prospect of receiving mail made me hopeful.

Three months into my prison stay, I received a letter from my lawyer. After much anticipation on my part, he couldn't confirm my release. It read: "I don't know when you will be released, but I know that it will be soon." It was a far cry from what I had expected.

Saddened and depressed, I reached for my second letter of that evening addressed from my mother. Inside were pictures of my younger sisters, cousins, and cancer-ridden grandfather. My elation was fleeting, however, as I realized that I shouldn't expect to see all the people I loved anytime soon.

Lifting my blanket over my head, I started to cry for the first time in the Texas State Penitentiary.

Crying in prison is a reputation killer. It's a recipe for disaster as a sign of weakness. Here I was whimpering under my blanket after less than three months of incarceration.

As I wept, my failures and embarrassments filled my head. I had stolen documents from a museum where I worked to pay for my tuition. My parents were deeply hurt, the financial toll cost my sisters their college fund, and there seemed to be no way out. I cried myself to sleep. This was my rock bottom moment.

After a moment like that, it's difficult to see a path to redemption. In retrospect, however, it was precisely the breakdown that I needed. From that point onward, a sense of surrender pervaded my prison experience. Rather than waiting desperately for mail and phone calls with my family, I crafted a routine and plan. If I was going to redeem myself, it had to start from within the prison cell, not when I was released.

I started with my habits. From prison, I had no access to nootropics or smart drugs. I could only change my lifestyle. First, I began doing calisthenics workouts and walking for hours every day. Then I stopped eating packages of cookies to salve my emotional pain.

Before long I was eating a diet high in healthy fish, protein, and vegetables—even within prison walls. In one instance, I purchased exorbitantly priced bell peppers and onions stolen by another inmate from the kitchen. I would do whatever it took to improve my mental and physical performance.

It worked. With the foundation of a healthy lifestyle, I stopped watching rerun TV and started reading books from the library. As my brain became sharper, I read nearly forty books over the next three months. It shifted my mindset and prepared me for release.

The most drastic changes I made in prison were achieved by altering my lifestyle and habits alone. By the end of my prison stay, I was able to focus for longer periods, creative ideas were flowing, my strength and muscle mass had grown, and my mood was fantastic.

There were no nootropics or smart drugs involved until after my release from prison. Dialing in these habits is the most important first step and is a significant aspect of this book.

If you have come looking for a book about the latest drugs, you're going to be disappointed. This book will teach you how to be more intelligent, focused, creative, and successful, but smart drugs are only a fraction of doing that. We must first start by optimizing all other aspects of our lives, such as sleep and diet.

Before we go any further, ask yourself why becoming more intelligent, focused, creative, and successful is important. For many, it's simply a way to make a lot of money. The more nootropics one takes, the better they can perform in their job and accumulate resources.

If financial gain is your only reason to learn about cognitive enhancement, this book includes plenty of tools and tricks, but you'll also find more meaningful approaches.

How to Use This Book

This book will explain how to approach cognitive enhancement. I will provide specific recommendations and action steps, but my goal is to help you think for yourself when analyzing brain optimization information elsewhere.

It is not an encyclopedia of nootropics or smart drugs. It is not a simple three-step method to improve mental performance, and it will provide no Limitless pill suggestions. Visit the resource page at *http://www.aheadabovebook.com/resources* for more clarity on these topics as they will not be here.

Even if I authored a book about all the different chemical substances and their respective benefits, science and technology change too rapidly. I want this book to be relevant for decades no matter the year.

So, while there is an entire section dedicated to nootropics and the methods that myself and experts use to increase mental performance, the primary purpose of this book is to teach you how to approach cognitive enhancement and nootropics so that you aren't overwhelmed or confused.

The book is split into two separate sections. One, entitled *Beyond the Pill*, discusses the many aspects that influence our cognitive abilities outside of nootropics or smart drugs.

This will include sleep, exercise, and dietary factors that affect cognitive abilities, but also other lesser-known contributors, such as evolutionary psychology, community, and positive psychology.

The foundation of this section is an evolutionary approach, which is why Native American tribes and behaviors will provide key take-aways for improving cognition.

In the second section covering nootropics, I'll discuss the chemical compounds themselves, but from a unique perspective.

For both of these sections, there are some essential ideas you must understand. Like building a new home, we must lay a sturdy foundation. If you skip everything else, make sure to read the following fundamental concepts.

THREE CORE CONCEPTS — OF — COGNITIVE ENHANCEMENT

#1. THE BRAIN-BODY CONNECTION

Summary: *Any attempt to optimize mental performance independent of the body is unsustainable. Take a complex systems approach by creating habits that optimize mind and body.*

When I was sixteen years old, having little experience with what girls liked or wanted, I wrote a poem for my high school crush. Whenever close to Sarah-Beth McDonald during chemistry class, my heart fluttered, my stomach flipped, and my throat tightened—and I felt like she needed to know that.

Seeing her rejection note the same day created a physical sensation most people have felt before. The sinking ache in the stomach and tension around the chest were a direct result of my emotions and feelings.

The fear and anxiety I associated with this rejection created a cascade of chemical reactions throughout my body and brain. The math quiz I failed that afternoon was the icing on the day's already terrible cake. And that big, red "F" probably wouldn't have happened had my heart not been broken hours before.

Our emotions and feelings directly impact our cognitive performance because our body and brain are connected.

The brain is the most complex object in the universe, and I'm not only talking about the piece between your ears.[8]

Neurons, or nerve cells, carry the brain's electrical "messages." Many of these connections pass through the brain stem and branch out to every region of the body. If you touch a hot stove, messages are being sent to the brain to indicate pain and heat quickly. Thanks to the brain-body connection, your hand will pull away long before you consciously determine you should do so.

Given the reciprocal relationship and rapid-fire communication happening between the brain and the body, is it any wonder that the health of each relies on the other? Or that optimizing the health of the body is essential for enhancing the brain's cognition?

Now, the idea of the brain-body connection may be easy to understand through the lens of a hand on a hot stove, but we're talking about 100 billion neurons with nearly infinite complexity. The idea is simple; the inner workings of your neural networks are not.

The complexity of the human system brings up two things:

---

8   Ira Flatow (Host). "Decoding 'the Most Complex Object in the Universe'" NPR News. June 14, 2013.

1. Cause and effect certainty
2. Emphasis of emotional health

When the difference in our memory, learning ability, or concentration can be caused by tens of thousands of various complex mechanisms, it is nearly impossible to have 100% certainty about causes and effects.

As I write this, approximately 300 mg of phenylpiracetam is passing through my bloodstream. I took the same dosage at the same time from the same bottle this morning as I have many other mornings, but this time it's been nearly two weeks since my last dose.

One would expect my tolerance to have gone away, but alas, today doesn't feel as stimulating as it has before, and I'm baffled. This experience occurs because there are so many variables and complexity within the human system.

Even with my years of experience and self-experimentation, I cannot be certain. This means we cannot jump to conclusions about whether something "works" or not based on a single anecdotal event. In my example, phenylpiracetam clearly works, but not in this specific instance.

The second factor is our emotional health, which is not often connected to cognitive performance. Feelings of depression, isolation, or anxiety are not conducive to optimal mental performance.

A nootropic will not counteract a painful emotional experience, such as losing a loved one, no matter how powerful it might be.

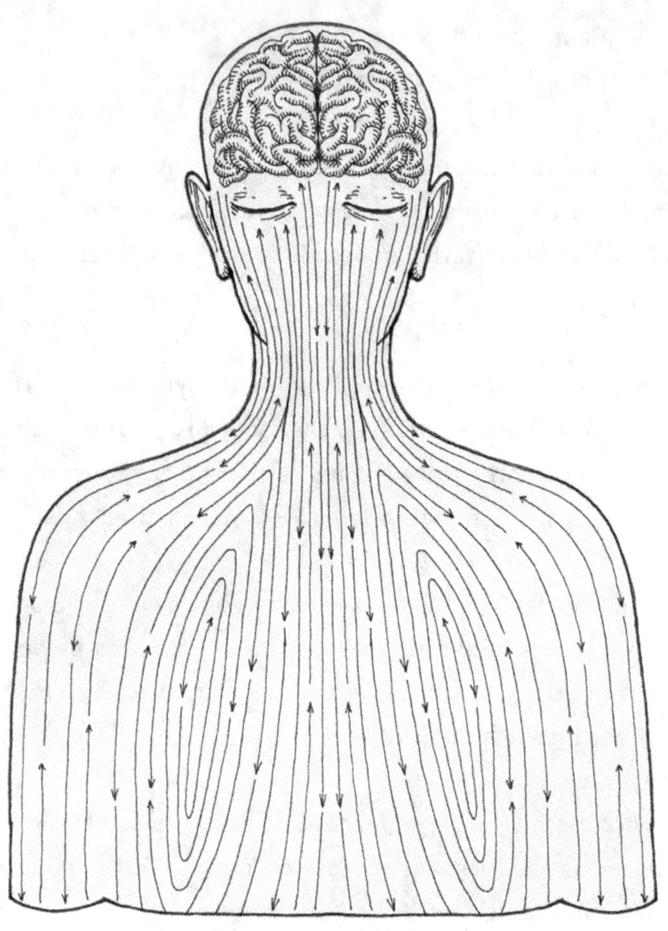

According to Dr. Wilhelm Reich, these negative emotions create subconscious physical patterns in our body. Tension across the chest may seem like a physical problem but is strongly correlated with emotional trauma.

During Reich's 20th century career, he founded a field of study called Bioenergetic analysis, which focused on the interconnectedness of the brain and the body. He would help clients "get into their body" by promoting dancing and other behaviors of physical expression, which has helped millions of people overcome mood disorders and fears over the past few decades.

If we ignore our body when optimizing our brain, we do so at our peril. In contrast to Reich's work, conventional wisdom states, "mind over matter," as if our brain has unlimited control over our body.

In reality, the brain and body are highly connected, and both require constant care and attention. If we want to optimize our mental performance, we cannot disregard the needs of the body.

#2. UNIQUE BRAIN CHEMISTRY

Summary: *Each individual is unique. Each day is unique. Cognitive enhancing techniques that work for one person do not work for others. Focus on what works specifically for you regardless of marketing hype or scientific analysis.*

Sitting across from friend and business owner Zach Obront, I sipped my green juice at the Whole Foods flagship in Austin, Texas. Explaining nootropics and cognitive enhancement, I asked whether Zach had tried supplementation.

"My dad and I purchased a dozen modafinil pills, but when I tried it, nothing happened..."

I was flummoxed. How could a nootropic compound so radically powerful for me have absolutely no impact on Zach?

Each individual has unique brain chemistry, which is individualized and specific. Not only is each person's brain chemistry unique compared to others, but may be unique depending on the phase of life or even time of day.

Human DNA is 99.9% the same, but within that fraction of a difference are many variations of the human experience. There are two main contributing factors to our unique brain chemistry:

1. Genetic factors
2. Environmental stimuli

Our genetic makeup plays a huge role on how cognitive enhancement and nootropics will impact our brain. In Zach's case, he may have what Dr. Bodenmann discovered as a Met/Met [A/A] genotype.[9]

This may not mean much, but it is a very specific gene expression that influences Zach's experience as a non-responder with modafinil.

For me, the experience is the opposite. Like many who have tried modafinil, it greatly impacts my workflow by adding focus, concentration, and clarity of mind. It's easy for me to see the big picture when taking modafinil, which is a far cry from Zach's lackluster experience.

---

9   S Bodenmann. "Pharmacogenetics of Modafinil After Sleep Loss: Catechol-O-Methyltransferase Genotype Modulates Waking Functions But Not Recovery Sleep ". *Nature*. Mar 2009. and Sereina Bodenmann. "Effects of Modafinil on the Sleep EEG Depend on Val158Met Genotype of COMT". *Sleep*. Aug 1, 2010.

Another common example is an MTHFR gene mutation (often jokingly referred to as the "motherfucker gene"), which afflicts 40% of the population.[10] The MTHFR is an enzyme that adds a methyl group to folic acid (vitamin B9) to make it usable in the body. Without having an essential vitamin like folate, many suffer from reduced cognitive performance, poor memory, lethargy, and lack of focus.

The co-founder of Paleo F(x), Keith Norris, discovered he had this mutation and began a simple supplement regimen including methylfolate (a simple, cheap supplement found in any grocery store) to get proper nutrition. Of course, getting this vital nutrient provided more benefits to him than the most cutting-edge nootropic.

If you're new to cognitive enhancement and nootropics, these genes might seem more complicated than they are. With a simple genetic test (currently around $100 to $200), anyone can learn about the two examples mentioned above.

The second factor influencing our unique brain chemistry is environmental stimuli, which includes our daily habits and lifestyle choices. A vegan would have unique brain chemistry compared to someone eating a Paleo-style diet. A vegan eating fewer eggs or meat might find supplemental choline and creatine are more useful than anything else.

Here is also where different lifestyle factors can change the unique brain chemistry on a day-to-day level.

---

10   Elizabeth Pennisi. ENCODE Project Writes Eulogy for Junk DNA. *Science*. Vol 337, 7 September 2012.

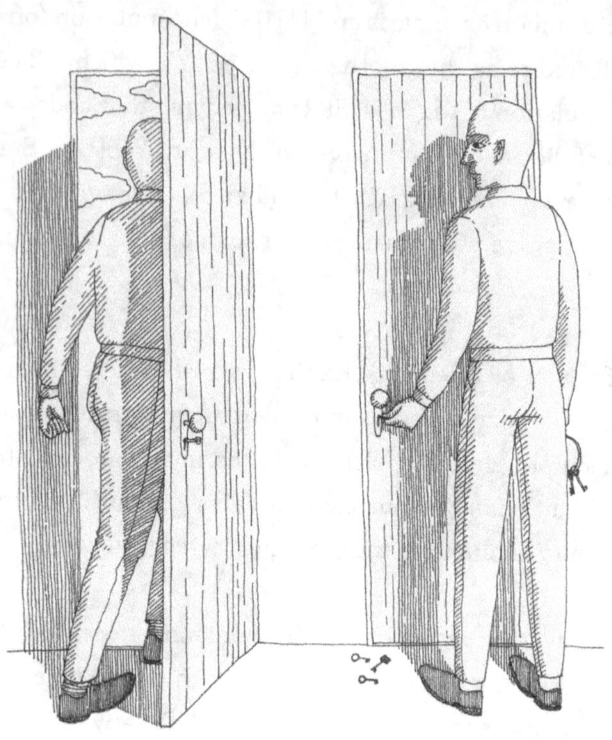

When I wake up refreshed from a full night of sleep, using a noo-tropic like modafinil (or even the caffeine and L-theanine combi-nation) is far more effective than days when I am sleep deprived. Same drug, different environmental changes.

Understanding the uniqueness of each brain is not a new concept. Doctor Eric Braverman was one of the pioneers in the field of indi-vidualized brains and treating them differently.

Over his four decades of experience and research at the Harvard Medical School, he has published numerous works including the popular book, *The Edge Effect*.

Within the book, Braverman provides a basic understanding of each individual's unique brain. The book includes a subjective True / False test that helps readers narrow down the causes of certain cognitive deficiencies. There are flaws with this test, but it is a good starting point. As our technology grows more robust, we will have quantitative data showing the uniqueness of our brain not once, but continuously and in real-time.

Why Does Uniqueness Matter?

Understanding the uniqueness of each brain allows us to achieve greater cognitive performance for a few reasons.

1. Finding strengths and reinforcing them
2. Identifying weaknesses and finding solutions

For genetic and environmental reasons, we have varying cognitive strengths and weaknesses. With a quick 23andme genetic test, Keith found that he struggled with an MTHFR gene mutation, making him unable to use vital nutrients properly. Once he identified the weakness, it was a fairly straightforward supplement tweak that made drastic cognitive improvements for him.

Learning the strengths of our unique brain from both genetic and environmental perspectives will also help us optimize further so that we do not trade one weakness for another.

Of course, uniqueness matters because it provides us power and self-responsibility. Sometimes it seems like health information not only changes constantly but it even contradicts itself.

Researchers and doctors (both of whom are more "expert" than we are) have varying opinions, and it may seem impossible to determine what is true.

With an understanding of the uniqueness of our brains, however, that is no longer the case. Researchers and doctors may know more about a particular topic and how it influences the society in general, *but not how it affects you specifically.*

In narrowing our scope to just our brain, not only do we avoid being swayed by another's' opinion or "facts," but we also prevent dogmatic belief in any particular nootropic or method of cognitive enhancement.

As the adage goes, someone without any vices is sure to have some annoying virtues. Dogma in cognitive enhancement isn't helpful. We must see each brain as unique based on both the person and the time.

My experience with fasting provides a perfect example. When first starting a fasting regimen, my experience was positive. Over time, fasting for at least sixteen hours per day became one of the best practices I could do for both my brain and body. It works great for me, popular biohackers like Tim Ferriss rave about it—but plenty of women see terrible results.

After speaking to woman after woman who tried a similar fasting regimen, it seemed obvious to me there was an element of uniqueness. For someone who has had a bad experience, all the science in the world will not (nor should it) be convincing.

You are in charge of your cognitive performance. Don't give up that responsibility to a doctor, to a friend, or even to me. As a unique individual, run experiments on yourself to determine what does and doesn't work for you.

#3. 80 / 20 RULE

Of your cognitive enhancement results, 80% will come from only 20% of your efforts.

The 80 / 20 rule, also known as the Pareto principle, is primarily a business law with applications to any system—from success to sports to software to the brain—and, in general, suggests that 80% of the effects are a result of 20% of the causes.

For the purposes of cognitive enhancement, adhering to this principle not only improves cognitive performance, it also provides a sustainable and enjoyable lifestyle.

Let's continue with our fasting example.

Fasting works for me and I'm a big proponent, but sometimes warmly baked, Icelandic pastries are too seductive and I'll break my fast early (and throw gluten-free out the window).

So long as I maintain my fasting regimen most of the time, I see tremendous benefits. In fact, fasting *most* of the time gives me benefit, while fasting *all* the time gives me marginal added benefits *with additional mental stress*. In the end, it's usually not worthwhile for me to adhere to my fasting schedule 100%.

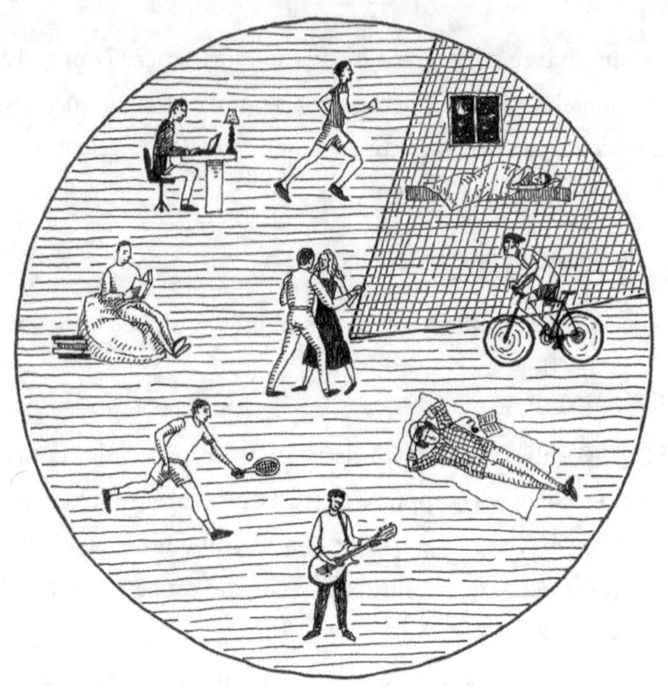

The same holds true for much of the advice on nootropics and cognitive enhancement that you will get throughout this book, online, and in other media resources.

There are thousands of biohacks, nootropics, and lifestyle changes that will give us a fraction of a percent better memory or focus. The irony of trying to follow all of this advice is that it hurts us in a few different ways:

1. Resource cost (time, money etc.)
2. Mental stress

Many of these techniques and lifestyle changes either cost a lot of money, or they consume hours of the day. Given that nootropics and cognitive enhancement are my full-time priority, profession, and passion, my morning routine consists of at least thirty to forty-five minutes of turning off my sleep tracking app, using my heart rate variability monitor, taking nootropics, and meditating.

Extrapolate that to include all of the various things we are told we "should" do in order to perform our best, and we wouldn't have time to do anything else. In the end, we would spend hours of precious time tracking and tweaking things simply to achieve higher cognitive performance without applying it to anything.

Beyond the loss of time and money, following too much cognitive enhancement advice can also lead to more stress. The idea that maintaining strict self-control and willpower draws from limited mental resources is called "ego depletion."[11]

According to research, any task requiring some measure of self-control can have a hindering effect on subsequent self-control tasks even if they're unrelated. Spending too much mental energy on improving cognitive enhancement could *hurt* your work and professional life.

The final irony of taking an obsessive approach to cognitive enhancement is the impact of stress on cognition. Any stress response will reduce cognitive performance in both the short and long term.[12]

---

11   Baumeister RF. "Ego depletion: is the active self a limited resource?" *J Pers Soc Psychol*. May 1998.

12   McEwen BS. "Stress and cognitive function." *Curr Opin Neurobiol*. April 1995.

If we're bashing our heads against the wall trying to keep up with every cognitive enhancement technique or nootropic drug, we're going to burn out and create far more problems than we solve.

BEYOND THE PILL

Every morning while in prison, fifty-three inmates woke up to bright lights and the sound of chow at 4:30 AM. A small fraction rubbed groggy eyes, put on orange jumpsuits and sandals, and shuffled towards the trays full of food.

I never ate at 4:30 in the morning because it disrupted my routine. With those same groggy eyes, I woke up, stashed away all the food into my bowls, and filled up a water bottle with the protein-filled rehydrated "milk" the cafeteria served.

Trying to maintain healthy practices in prison was difficult. If I had my way, things would have been much different. Although I wish I had better habits and access to healthier foods while incarcerated, my experience showed me that our daily choices are more important than anything else.

Simply making the right diet, exercise, and mindset choices in prison was enough to shift my experience even when I had no nootropics or smart drugs to push me in the right direction. Any prisoner will admit that achieving success within the confines of prison requires creativity and resourcefulness.

Maybe you don't want to spend hundreds of dollars on supplements that don't work. Maybe you don't need high-powered stimulants to achieve your goals. In this section, I'll show you how to achieve an optimal level of cognitive performance by focusing on your habits and lifestyle choices alone.

Keeping in mind the three fundamental concepts outlined in the introduction, we'll tackle four specific areas of our lives that influence cognition without any pills, drugs, or supplements.

This section is broken down as such:

1. **Mindset** – How we view the world and our place in it.
2. **Relationships** – Our feeling of interconnectedness with people in our lives.
3. **Diet** – The fuel we use to power our brains.
4. **Lifestyle** – The habits filling our day that help or hurt our cognitive performance.

MINDSET

"Can you explain why you believe prison was the best thing that ever happened to you?" questioned Kimberly Rich during our podcast interview.

The challenge of my six-month prison experience gave me a taste of hardship, which helped me to grow into a more mature, confident, and driven individual.

 It shifted my mindset and allowed me to view the world through a different lens, one that most upper-middle class individuals may never see. Once I had been there, learned my lessons, and brought them back to the real world, there was no going back.

After over five years involved with nootropics and cognitive enhancement, I cannot count the number of people who have asked me how they can become more motivated, how to create a "Limitless Mindset," or how to stop procrastinating.

All of these inquiries have little to do with specific nootropics or biohacks, and everything to do with mindset changes. They may be asking a nootropics expert for help from a drug, but what they really seek is a change in their mindset.

With the right mindset towards life, challenges, and completing fulfilling work, much is possible. Those with determination find a way; gratitude is the happiness equalizer, and patience is a virtue.

Our conversation about mindset will be purely pragmatic. Modern research consistently proves how our mindset shapes our actions and our results. Now we can view how gratitude changes our brain waves or how flow enhances learning. We'll start with why humans do everything because our highest biological priority influences many aspects of cognition and our lives.

Why We Do Everything

From a biological perspective, any species has but one focus or goal to achieve throughout their life: *reproduction*. All animals (including humans) strive to pass on their genes and unique DNA to the next generation. The more copies the better so long as they can survive to pass on their DNA as well.

Of course, if our body's objective is to reproduce and pass on our DNA, our psychology and mindset will shift accordingly. This field of study, evolutionary psychology, is relatively new, but well-founded and researched.

Evolutionary psychology becomes vitally important for understanding everything from the type of brain one has to our level of creativity and capabilities. It is not a stretch to say that our cognitive performance is directly linked to our evolved psychological behaviors.

One prime example is called the "age-genius curve." Studies of male jazz musicians, painters, writers, and scientists suggest all perform their best in their early adulthood (20-30's) and then their professional performance begins to fade.[13]

---

13   Satoshi Kanazawa. 2003. "Why Productivity Fades with Age: The Crime Genius Connection." *Journal of Research in Personality.* 37: 257 - 72

Male scientists who never get married continue publishing papers throughout their life, approximately 50% in young adulthood and 50% in later life. In contrast, male scientists who do get married unconsciously signal that they are passing their genes and DNA. They publish 95.8% of their best work before marriage and only 4.2% afterward.[14]

Evolutionary psychology is a prime example of how our conscious desires can be less important than millions of years of biology. If we allow the whims of our biology to dictate our behavior, we will end up performing poorly, unhappy, and unsuccessful. It's not that we must fight our nature, but recognize its existence so that we can adapt accordingly.

Understanding that our brains are different for evolutionary reasons gives us guidance for our strengths and weaknesses. Of course, one of the great equalizers is a psychological phenomenon humans have evolved called "flow."

Dropping Into Flow

Male or female, one thing all humans have in common is the flow state. Our Greek ancestors believed flow came from the "Muse," an inspirational goddess involved with all works of art.

Over the past few decades, research on flow states in the brain has amplified our understanding and the ease of replicating this phenomenon.

---

14   Satoshi Kanazawa. 2000. "Scientific Discoveries as Cultural Displays: A Further Test of Miller's Courtship Model." *Evolution and Human Behavior*. 21: 317-21.

According to the pioneer, Mihály Csíkszentmihályi, flow is a mental state in which the person performing an activity is fully immersed, creating a sense of enjoyment, focus, and clarity. Often referred to as "getting in the zone," nearly any professional has experience with a similar feeling at some point in their lives.

The benefits of flow states are:

1.   Enhanced learning ability
2.   Increased creativity
3.   Improved focus (hyperfocus)

When flow researchers Jamie Wheal and Steven Kotler visited the Google headquarters, they measured technology that tracked the heart rate and brain patterns of the company's founders. When Google co-founder Sergey Brin used the "looping swing" (a device created to induce flow), his brain and heart registered off-the-chart flow states associated with higher learning and creativity.[15]

Further research at Advanced Brain Monitoring in Carlsbad, California, suggested that an artificially induced flow state could cut down the training time novice snipers required to become experts by up to 50%.

Compare these novice snipers who increased learning by up to 50% with similar memory-enhancing nootropic drugs (such as piracetam). One of the few piracetam studies shows only an 8.6%

---

15   Steven Kotler and Jamie Wheal. *Stealing Fire: How Silicon Valley, the Navy SEALs, and Maverick Scientists are Revolutionizing the Way We Live and Work*. Pg. 385.

increase in memory formation.[16] Often, as is the case with flow, there are better places to commit our resources than buying a pill.

Beyond learning ability, flow has applications for creativity. Most researchers believe creativity is related to our working memory. Essentially, it's our ability to hold many different ideas and combine them to create new solutions.

Australian researchers tested flow and creativity by creating a challenging brain teaser and asking participants to solve it. Under normal circumstances, no participants could solve the teaser. When the researchers induced a flow state artificially, nearly 40% of the participants could solve the puzzle.

Steven Kotler and Jamie Wheal have conducted one of the largest flow experiments through Kotler's Flow Genome Project and found people were 6 to 8 times more creative while in a flow state.

In the world of nootropics and cognitive enhancement, one of the most common questions I see is "how do I increase creativity?" Few substances have an impact on creativity, but flow states are a ready solution.

Finally, there is a sense of hyperfocus associated with flow states. This isn't always considered a good thing (it's why people play video games for hours without end), but in the context of our professional lives, it can be highly useful.

---

16   Dimond SJ. "Increase in the power of human memory in normal man through the use of drugs." *Psychopharmacology*. Sep 29,1976.

One of the main features of flow states is the ability to block out nearly everything going on in the environment. This freedom from distraction is often produced from brain chemicals, such as dopamine and adrenaline, which are similar to caffeine and other concentration nootropics (though less substantial).

The same chemical compounds create effects in the brain whether they come endogenously (from within the body, such as a flow state) or exogenously (from outside the body, such as a nootropic or smart drug).

There is a final cognitive benefit to flow, which has impacted Steven Kotler personally. Flow states can enhance immune health and reduce autoimmune deficiencies.

Before Kotler studied and wrote about flow states, he struggled with debilitating Lyme disease.

"I was going to kill myself because all I was going to be from that point on was a burden to my friends and family. I was not a functioning human being at all..." recounts Kotler.[17]

When a persistent friend insisted on surfing for the day, a skeptical Kotler acquiesced and headed to Sunset Beach in Los Angeles, California, struggling all the while.

Although nearly unable to walk, he remembered: "...I feel great. I feel better than I've felt in three years. My muscles don't hurt. I'm clear headed. It was astounding, quasi-mystical."

---

17   Steven Kotler interview with Dave Asprey. Episode #109.

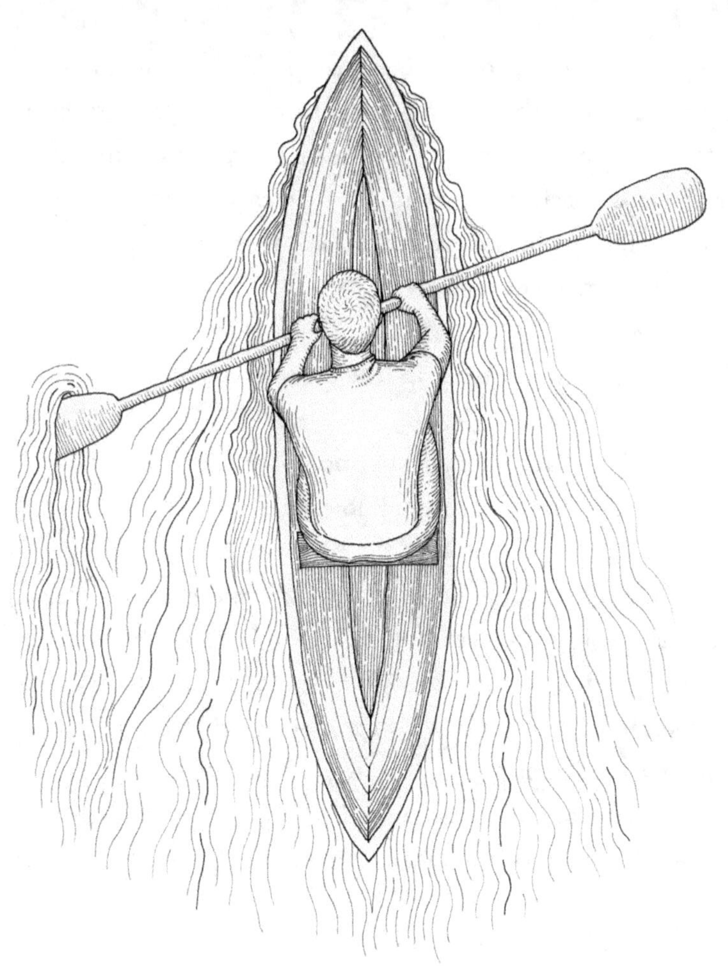

Kotler continued surfing over the next six months, despite needing fourteen days to recover. He went from functioning around 10% capacity up to 80% and started researching why surfing was providing such results.

He found that flow states amplify immune strength. The neurochemicals associated with flow help to reset the nervous system, while stress chemicals like cortisol and norepinephrine get flushed out.

Flow states are one of the few sustainable mental states we can achieve to enhance our cognitive performance in a long-term way. Our task is to bring this psychological phenomenon into our lives as often as possible to produce more creative, focused, and effective work. Most have experienced a flow state before, but how do we reverse engineer them?

There are two ways we can induce more flow into our lives.

1. Chemical combinations and nootropics
2. Organizing life around flow states

The chemically induced flow states work sometimes but they aren't long-term solutions. According to Steven Kotler, one way to induce an artificial flow state is by drinking a cup of coffee (dopamine and adrenaline), going for a walk (producing endorphins), and then smoking marijuana (THC).[18] Now you're ready to tackle challenging problems because this combination mimics the chemicals of a flow state. Be aware, though, that it will not be effective for long.

The second method of inducing more flow into our lives is what researcher Cal Newport considers "deep work." This is the ability to focus without distraction on a cognitively demanding task, and it is one of the most effective cognitive enhancers we can use.

Deep Work to Flow

The ultimate path to flow states, increased learning, creativity, and better work is "deep work": uninterrupted, distraction-free work on

---

18   Steven Kotler interview with Joe Rogan. November 2016.

the things that matter in your personal or professional life."[19]

While most applicable in the professional world, deep work can be a period of intense focus on artwork or any other meaningful task that brings fulfillment. It is intrinsically beneficial for life satisfaction, but the resulting chemical changes to the brain also provide significant cognitive enhancement benefits.

Deep work triggers activity in the prefrontal cortex in regions associated with cognition, emotion, maintenance of internal goals, and reward circuitry. Regions of the brain that activate during periods of "boredom" were less active during this mental state.[20]

There are two barriers to achieving deep work in our lives:

1. Consistent stimulation
2. Poor brain recovery

Our brains are wired to anticipate novel stimuli in our environment. According to Dr. Clifford Nass, a researcher at Stanford:

"Throughout evolutionary history, a big surprise would get everyone's brain thinking...But we've got a large and growing group of people who think the slightest hint that something interesting might be going on is like catnip. They can't ignore it."[21]

---

19   Cal Newport. *Deep Work: Rules for Focused Success in a Distracted World*.

20   Yoshida K. "Brain activity during the flow experience: a functional near-infrared spectroscopy study." *Neurosci Lett*. June 24, 2014.

21   Matt Richtel. "Attached to Technology and Paying a Price". *New York Times*. JUNE 6, 2010.

Research by Nass and other scientists have found that modern things like email and social media over-stimulate our brains. Not only does this cause more stress, it also wires our brains differently than our ancestors.[22]

Imagine a scenario that has probably played out thousands of times: I'm sitting at the computer, preparing to complete a project. Then cursor moves to open a new tab. Automatically typing, the browser brings up Facebook before I realize what has happened.

Once I come to my senses, it's too late. The small red buttons offering notifications and unread messages provide small squirts of dopamine in my brain. With consistent social media and email, our brains become rewired. They crave the dopamine and neurochemical changes that keep us addicted and unable to complete deep work.[23]

In combination with unlimited supplies of savory, sweet, and fatty foods (all providing rewarding and addicting brain chemicals), our entire lifestyle becomes geared towards craving dopamine and away from deep work.

It is unsurprising that nearly 60% of the questions I receive about nootropics and cognitive enhancement are related to improved focus and concentration. We would like to believe there is an easy solution—a pill or smart drug for unlimited focus and

---

22   Gloria Mark. "The Cost of Interrupted Work: More Speed and Stress". University of California, Irvine.

23   Mauri M. "Why is Facebook so successful? Psychophysiological measures describe a core flow state while using Facebook." *Cyberpsychol Behav Soc Netw*. Dec 2011.

concentration—but often our attention span is a sum total of small tasks and habits like social media.

The answer to this over-stimulation is as Cal Newport explains: *boredom*. The more comfortable we become with boredom in our daily life, the greater the likelihood we will be able to concentrate on the things that really matter.

An example Newport gives is waiting in line and pulling out our smartphones. In line, we have nothing to do physically; we can only remain patient. Because our smartphones are chock full with small dopamine spurts, we choose to access them and shut boredom out. Next time (even if you do it once), opt for cringe-worthy boredom instead.

The more we can train our brain to be okay with boredom, the easier deep work becomes. Even in the late 19th century, Henry David Thoreau felt over-stimulated and distracted by his New England compatriots.

Thoreau sought the solace of Walden Pond, where he wrote for nearly four years. It's no wonder that Thoreau produced some of his best work during this period; he was practicing long periods of deep work and becoming accustomed to boredom.

Of course, the lifestyle changes I advocate are more modest than Thoreau's. There is no need to renounce earthly pleasures, live the monk's life, or move to a pasture to achieve more deep work.

One simple alternative is to use tools and technology that free us from distraction rather than foster it. This includes airplane mode on our phones, turning off email notifications, and installing the Facebook "newsfeed killer" Chrome application.

While email and social media can allow us to remain connected and in communication with friends, we can take steps to avoid becoming inundated with news, cat videos, and other distractions we would be prone to consuming. We can more easily organize our lives around periods of deep work to optimize our cognitive performance.

The less obstructive, though equally problematic reason we struggle with deep work is our lack of mental recovery.

Deep work is not meant to last long periods. According to researcher Anders Ericsson, novices can only perform uninterrupted deep work around one hour per day, while experts manage only four hours.

As a culture, we reward many hours of shallow work instead of these few hours of deep work. Entrepreneurs and startups often glamorize 80 hour work weeks. Professional, salaried employees are forced to contribute a minimum of eight hours per day.

Most of the time, replying to emails, scheduling meetings and calls are considered "shallow work" and do little to advance whatever project we're most trying to achieve. Yet these trivial tasks fill up our day and make it impossible for the brain to recover.

As mentioned in the core concepts section, our brain has finite mental resources, which run out (ego depletion). If we perform any kind of deep work, these mental resources may run out even quicker.

The theory of ego depletion is studied in a psychology setting, but zooming into the biochemistry provides similar conclusions. The brain communicates using neurotransmitters, which are finite unless we afford the time to replenish them.[24]

The answer is to disconnect from work and mentally taxing tasks daily to allow our brain to adequately replenish various chemicals, so it does not interfere with deep work and flow of the next day.

Many well-intentioned professionals answer emails and perform work duties until the moment they go to sleep. Not only is this less enjoyable rest time, it also negatively impacts our ability to perform deep work the next day. Instead, set firm boundaries that allow adequate replenishment for your brain.

At my home, smartphones routinely go on airplane mode in the early evening. My friends and business colleagues have no way of reaching me even if they tried, which may seem isolationist, but helps me to disconnect from distracting technology and focus on what is most important.

Unfortunately, these two barriers to deep work are not mutually exclusive. The same person who might check Facebook a hundred and thirty times in one day may also respond to work emails at 11:30 PM before going to bed. Both of them are barriers to deep

---

24   This is especially true when using nootropics or smart drugs, which alter the amount or rate of usage of these vital chemicals.

work, which limits not only our cognitive capacity but also our satisfaction.

Engaging in deep work doesn't require a significant expenditure of time, but the investment is worthwhile. Kotler's research (and a ten-year McKinsey study[25]) suggests flow increases productivity by at least five times. Better work in less time. Flow is cognitive enhancement at its finest, and without a single chemical compound.

An Attitude of Gratitude

"Does that mean that we can be grateful for everything? Certainly not. We cannot be grateful for violence, for war, for oppression, for exploitation. On the personal level, we cannot be grateful for the loss of a friend, for unfaithfulness, for bereavement. But I didn't say we can be grateful for everything. I said we can be grateful in every given moment for the opportunity..."

—DAVID STEINDL-RAST, BENEDICTINE MONK

In June 2014, the Greater Good Science Center at the University of California at Berkeley launched phase one of their well-funded (tens of millions) project called "Expanding the Science and Practice of Gratitude."

Their self-described objective is to promote evidence-based practices of gratitude in medical, educational, and organizational settings. The aim isn't only to increase positive moods and feelings but

---

25 Susie Cranston. "Increasing the 'meaning quotient' of work" *McKinsey Quarterly*. January 2013.

to make substantive biochemical changes. For example, gratitude can improve sleep quality and reduce blood pressure.[26]

The concept of being grateful for cognitive enhancement purposes may seem outlandish, but there are few scientific institutions more well-respected than the University of California. Nonetheless, understanding of how gratitude influences the brain is in its infancy.

To date, only two studies utilize brain scans (fMRI) to detect changes during or after periods of gratitude.

One published in *Frontiers of Psychology* noted that regions of the brain associated with moral cognition, value judgment, and theory of mind[27] were influenced by gratitude practices.[28]

The other provided a more solid understanding of gratitude as it impacts cognitive performance. The study concluded that a simple gratitude practice (e.g., listing things one is grateful for) could help rewire the brain even up to three months later.[29]

The participants of the study were undergoing counseling as part of treatment for anxiety and depression. At the two-week mark,

---

26   Jackowska M. "The impact of a brief gratitude intervention on subjective well-being, biology and sleep." *J Health Psychol*. Oct 2016.

27   Theory of mind is essentially empathy. It is the ability to attribute mental states to oneself and understand that others have beliefs, perspectives, and desires that are different than one's own.

28   Fox GR. "Neural correlates of gratitude." *Front Psychol*. Sep 30,2015.

29   Kini P. "The effects of gratitude expression on neural activity." *Neuroimage*. Mar 2016.

many patients experienced greater satisfaction, but the longer-term three-month results were even more surprising.

Perhaps most interesting is the type of brain activity these patients showed during their gratitude practice. The neural pathways experienced when practicing gratitude were distinct and different from similar feelings of empathy, which suggests gratitude is a unique emotion.

The psychological changes of gratitude have been far more studied than the neurobiology, and results remain similar with focuses on two areas:

1. Reduced anxiety and depression
2. Improved mood and quality of life

In the world of nootropics and cognitive enhancement, one of the primary mechanisms of improving cognitive performance (test scores, cognition, etc.) is by reducing anxiety. This is how drugs like bacopa monnieri and others influence cognition.

Therefore, gratitude practices (and the rewiring that occurs as a result) can significantly influence cognitive performance with a mechanism similar to popular nootropics like bacopa monnieri.

Famed psychologist, Martin Seligman, contributed evidence that a single act of gratitude could reduce depressive symptoms by up to 35%. While these feelings faded over time, consistent gratitude practices provided more modest, but longer-term improvements.[30]

---

30   Seligman ME. "Positive psychology progress: empirical validation of interventions." *Am Psychol*. Jul-Aug 2005.

Compare that with some nootropics or even prescription drugs with anti-anxiety effects, and there isn't a huge difference. Of course, many of the available smart drugs have stronger biochemical effects than gratitude, but as these studies show, mindset matters as much as short-term chemical changes, if not more.

Increased time spent in a positive mood increases our quality of life. Seligman showed how a single act of gratitude could increase the quality of life by up to 10%.[31] This results from less envy and less materialism, both fulfilling ways to live. Gratitude is inherently beneficial for our mood.

Unlike the fleeting feeling of happiness, which can become burdensome when it dissipates, gratitude is applicable anywhere. It's difficult to be happy while in pain, but far easier to be grateful.

Over two years ago, while languishing in prison, I started a gratitude journal. Sitting in a cell was an experience that deeply shaped my perspective because it was so humbling. I was raised upper middle class and suddenly I had nothing. Even from that spot, I could be grateful for warm clothing and food. I found gratitude for countless books that I read and for the occasional letter from my family while incarcerated.

The practice is a simple one. I recommend jotting down a few things you are grateful for in a journal, on the notes app on your phone, or even a scrap piece of paper. Here are a few ideas:

____

31   Seligman ME. "Positive psychology progress: empirical validation of interventions." *Am Psychol*. Jul-Aug 2005.

1. Who are the friends and family who support you and in what way?
2. Where do you live and what luxuries does that afford you?
3. What education level have you achieved and how does this help?

The beauty of a practice like this is the self-perpetuating benefits of gratitude. Being grateful begets more gratitude. The list gets longer the more you do it.

Of course, the practice of gratitude takes many shapes and forms. Many Christians find it rewarding to note gratitude for their meals (saying grace). If writing isn't your thing, speak it aloud before eating with family.

However we choose to incorporate gratitude into our lives, it has long-standing cognitive effects. Not only do we engage otherwise dormant regions of our brains, but we do so for the long term. Gratitude isn't just a psychological phenomenon, but a biochemical one, too, and it can be on the magnitude of any smart drug or supplement.

As psychological research has flourished in the past century, we understand how influential our mindset can be. More than simply tricking yourself into believing, brain imaging techniques have confirmed real changes in the brain attributed to psychological practices. It's no surprise the best minds are taking full use of their mindset to achieve more.

RELATIONSHIPS

Humans are social animals. Like any other mammals, humans congregate into tribes and communities for protection, for education, and social bonding. The modern western economy and lifestyle are often opposed to our ancestral and community environments. As with eating a more ancestral diet (which we'll discuss later), having more "ancestral relationships," close ties to family and a network of friends, will have drastic cognitive effects.

Social isolation leads to increased stress chemicals, like cortisol, while strong interpersonal bonding enhances chemicals like oxytocin, prolactin, and vasopressin.[32]

Each of these bonding chemicals has unique benefits. Oxytocin deficiency is correlated with bipolar disorder, schizophrenia, and depression,[33] while more of this chemical is associated with physical touch and bonding, which can increase feelings of well-being.[34] Vasopressin, when derived naturally from social bonding, can enhance mental clarity, attention to detail, and short-term memory.[35][36]

---

32   Carter CS. "Neuroendocrine perspectives on social attachment and love." *Psychoneuroendocrinology*. Nov 1998.

33   David Cochran, MD, PhD. "The role of oxytocin in psychiatric disorders: A review of biological and therapeutic research findings." *Harv Rev Psychiatry*. Sep-Oct 2013.

34   Uvnäs-Moberg K. "Oxytocin may mediate the benefits of positive social interaction and emotions." *Psychoneuroendocrinology*. Nov 1998.

35   Millar K. "Vasopressin and memory: improvement in normal short-term recall and reduction of alcohol-induced amnesia." *Psychol Med*. May 1987.

36   Vawter MP. "Vasopressin fragment, AVP-(4-8), improves long-term and short-term memory in the hole board search task." *Neuropeptides*. Oct 1997.

The irony is, within nootropics and smart drug communities, there are biohackers who supplement with vasopressin and oxytocin but don't spend time building relationships and bonding socially.

No matter what nootropic we take, it will not replace our innate need for social bonding. Working for days on end without much interpersonal connection will reduce mental performance and increase cognitive burnout over time.

Examples of this are evident throughout the history of America. From the early days, Benjamin Franklin lamented the number of white European settlers joining Indian tribes with few Native Americans doing the opposite.[37] Any white settlers who spent time with tribal natives would "...take the first good opportunity of escaping again into the woods."

For hundreds of years, white European settlers sought the communal life of native tribes. Not for increased resources or comforts (tribal settings were often far more violent and harsh), but for the community aspects.

The famous Quanah Parker, considered the "Last Chief of the Comanche," was born to a white European mother named Cynthia Ann Parker. Despite being kidnapped at a young age, Parker was relocated to white settlements and spent the rest of her life trying to escape back to her Comanche tribe.[38]

---

37   Letters from Benjamin Franklin to Peter Collinson. Dated 9 May 1753.

38   Gwynne, S. C. (2010), *Empire of the Summer Moon*.

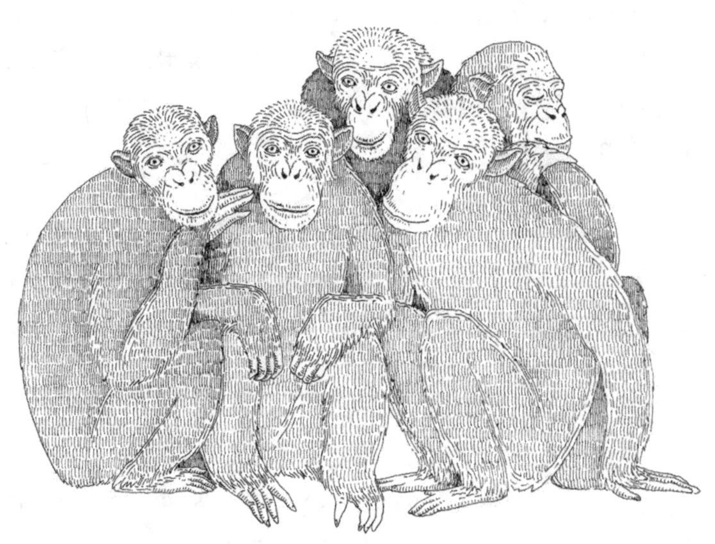

The Native American tribal experience came with violence and plenty of despair, but along with those characterizations was a strong sense of community. That same community aspect is largely gone from our modern, westernized, and highly individualized society.

Even today there are examples of this playing out in modern suburbia and urban environments. High rates of depression and anxiety are a direct result of poor interpersonal connection and a lack of the brain chemicals the human animal needs. A 2006 study of women in Nigeria, Canada, and the United States found that the most wealthy subset (American women) were the most depressed.[39]

---

39   Colla J. "Depression and modernization: a cross-cultural study of women." *Soc Psychiatry Psychiatr Epidemiol.* Apr 2006.

In fact, as economic resources are more plentiful, we become more anxious and depressed.[40] It isn't the wealth or resources that make us unhappy, but the lack of interpersonal relationships that accompanies it.

Today we have an even more distorted view of relationships. Instead of spending time with friends and family, we connect with people on Instagram and Facebook. This may provide some temporary relief, but it isn't true connection and provides few of the brain chemicals we need.

Interpersonal relationships are worthy investments of our time if we desire to optimize our cognitive performance.

When is the last time you remember feeling truly happy and fulfilled? Imagine the setting in detail. Perhaps you were with friends enjoying a few drinks, on a family vacation, or enjoying a meal with someone special. More than likely, our most happy moments involve other people.

Adding more connection into our lives does not need to be difficult or counterproductive. There is no need to join a commune, a cult, or tribe to receive adequate doses of the brain chemicals mentioned above. Instead, simply find a group of like-minded individuals in order to connect.

One of the most rewarding projects I've embarked upon is called "Intentional Dinners." Within these dinners, numerous (and

---

40   Brandon H Hidaka. "Depression as a disease of modernity: explanations for increasing prevalence." *J Affect Disord*. Nov 2012.

different) friends are invited to bring five random ingredients to cook with strangers for the evening tapas style. Each group takes turns cooking different foods, sharing, and discussing topics such as our greatest challenges, hopes, etc.

If this seems like overkill, try baby steps instead. We can incorporate more one-on-one time with friends in our social circle during the week. Looking online for meet-up groups can help bring like minded individuals together. Whatever the case may be, find opportunities to connect with others and interact on a more personal level.

Even for those of us who do not resonate with feeling depressed or anxious, reducing stress chemicals like cortisol will generally lead to better cognition, enhanced mental performance, and more fulfillment as well.

Family Matters

Our families all have flaws, but the family unit is one of the most important relationships one can foster. Not only are many of the above-mentioned brain chemicals associated predominantly with family, most people reading this book are at the tail end of their time together.

Writer Tim Urban calculated and wrote an impactful post detailing how much time he'll spend with his parents and siblings.[41]

"It turns out that when I graduated from high school, I had already

---

41   Tim Urban. "The Tail End" December 11, 2015.

used up 93% of my in-person parent time. I'm now enjoying the last 5% of that time," said Urban.

With similar assumptions, he reckoned time with his sisters was in the last 15%. These are estimates and will vary by person, but understanding how little time we have with our closest family members helps us to take better care of these relationships.

Living far away from loved ones may have perks financially or career-wise, but if it creates a feeling of isolation with resulting anxiety and depression, it's not worth it.

In the 1930s, Harry Harlow founded a rhesus monkey colony to study social isolation and the long-term effects it has on our primate ancestors. Early on, Harlow found that social isolation created a host of cognitive downsides, of which humans also suffer. The monkeys deprived of family time exhibited greater fear, anxiety, and anger throughout their life.

Since Harlow's initial experiments, cognitive scientists have found many correlations between isolation and mental performance using brain imaging technology. One study cited long-term memory deficits and decreased learning ability, which persisted even when monkeys were reunited with friends and family.[42]

In addition to cognitive performance, family bonding may correlate with longevity. In 2004, demographic researchers found communities in Sardinia, Italy, with an abundance of centenarians

---

42   Sánchez MM. "Differential rearing affects corpus callosum size and cognitive function of rhesus monkeys." *Brain Res*. Nov 23, 1998.

(people living beyond 100 years old). This study and their communities were the basis of Dan Buettner's book *Blue Zones*, which focused on five geographic areas of the world where people live the longest. He outlined nine unique traits of these communities, one of which is family bonding. In fact, a follow-up study found all the centenarians in Sardinia lived in a family home mostly with relatives.[43]

Family matters. When we prioritize our family and the quality time we spend with them, it sustainably alters a wide array of brain chemicals. We enhance our cognitive function, and we have more fulfilling and meaningful lives as well.

Humans have lived in small tribes for most of our species' history. For most of this time we were in intimate contact with both our immediate family, but also many friends and close contacts within the tribe. In contrast, many city-dwelling westerners live far away from their family and are surrounded by strangers rather than friends. It's not only damaging for our mood and happiness, but it harms our cognitive abilities. When we spend more time in contact with the people closest to us, it creates more fulfillment and allows us to better complete meaningful work.

------

43   Sonya Vasto. "Centenarians and diet: what they eat in the Western part of Sicily." *Immun Ageing*. 2012.

DIET

As evolution dictates our behavior so does it influence our ideal diet. Many specific diets have grown in popularity including Atkins, Ketogenic, and others. While these may help solve acute health symptoms and all have some merits, their complexity is not required for optimal mental performance.

Imagine a Lamborghini barreling down the road at ninety miles per hour. This finely tuned engine is both awe-inspiring and complex. Fickle in its taste, anything less than the highest quality fuel can cause long-term damage to the inner workings of the automobile.

If we were to fill our Lamborghini with a mixture of gasoline and manure, it wouldn't get far. We'd disrupt the engine, destroy the car, and pay a hefty price.

The same can be said for our brain. Although many people supplement with nootropics and smart drugs, most of our brain chemistry is altered by raw materials in our food. Provide the wrong kinds of food, and our brain won't perform optimally.

Instead of another complex diet, I believe in eating like we did two- to twelve-thousand years ago: not too much and fasting often. As we'll explore below, a healthy combination of these rules makes ancestral eating straightforward and sustainable while also prioritizing cognitive performance.

Fast for Freedom

Our ancestors lived a fascinating lifestyle. Before the agricultural revolution, they spent an average of two to four hours per day gathering food for themselves and the tribe. Often males would go on extended hunting trips, trekking through long stretches of unfamiliar terrain for a simple meal.

The Plains Native American tribes, virtually untouched by agriculture until European influence, were avid buffalo hunters and perfect examples of pre-agricultural societies. Comanche natives would spend days on the hunt, strategizing how to run these creatures off a cliff or pierce the thick hide with arrows and spears.

Food was sometimes plentiful, but often scarce. Fasting intermittently wasn't a fad diet, but rather a regular part of life.[44]

Over generations, our hunter-gatherer ancestors evolved to fast as part of their internal cleanup process, but with the increased food abundance that came with agricultural development, we have moved away from this habit. Humans were evolved to fast even though most do not.

Today, food is now ubiquitous and far more delicious. There are more calories for sale on every street corner than existed in an entire ancestral tribal village.

Excess calories create a cascade of consequences for the brain. First, our bodies never have an opportunity to look for cellular

44   Mark P. Mattson. "Meal frequency and timing in health and disease." *Proc Natl Acad Sci U S A*. Nov 25, 2014.

waste (a process called autophagy). Under normal fasting circumstances, this process essentially "takes out the trash" within our cells. If we are continually eating, the cells never have an opportunity to clean house.

This leads to neurodegeneration of the brain[45] and can have longer-term effects with relation to cancer and chronic diseases. In animal models, fasting can reduce the likelihood of certain cancer types.[46] In fact, a meta-analysis of fifty-nine fasting-related studies found 90.9% of the studies concluded fasting to have an anticancer role.[47]

Beyond cancer and neurodegeneration (both useful, but not cognitive *enhancement* per se), fasting has brain chemical shifts that can boost mental performance. One called brain-derived neurotrophic factor (BDNF) is associated with increased synaptic plasticity and neurogenesis.[48]

This may account for the increased memory formation and learning, which is often associated with an intermittent fasting regimen.[49]

---

45   Alirezaei M. "Short-term fasting induces profound neuronal autophagy." *Autophagy*. Aug 2010.

46   Brandhorst S. "Fasting and Caloric Restriction in Cancer Prevention and Treatment." *Recent Results Cancer Res*. 2016.

47   Mengmeng Lv. "Roles of Caloric Restriction, Ketogenic Diet and Intermittent Fasting during Initiation, Progression and Metastasis of Cancer in Animal Models: A Systematic Review and Meta-Analysis" *PLoS ONE*. December 11, 2014.

48   Valter D. Longo. "Fasting: Molecular Mechanisms and Clinical Applications." *Cell Metab*. Feb 4, 2014.

49   Liaoliao Li. "Chronic Intermittent Fasting Improves Cognitive Functions and Brain Structures in Mice." *PLoS One*. 2013.

Fasting offers us an opportunity to improve our cognitive performance by *removing* things from our lives rather than adding. For those who aren't looking to overcomplicate, like me, this is a perfect combination to help maintain my compliance and sanity.

What's even better about fasting is how simple it makes life. There may be situations where modern responsibilities restrict our time allocated to cooking or eating. With fasting, we can forego food, dishwashing, and maintain high cognitive output all the while.

Even with the data, I'm sure there are skeptical readers, and I can sympathize. My mother is the spokesperson for avoiding fasting at all costs.

"There is no way I can survive that many hours," she complains.

Then she bargains: "How about just twelve hours? I can do twelve hours."

If either of these sounds familiar, I've got good news. Any skeptics about fasting will only suffer from hunger pains for a few weeks. A hormone called ghrelin is the main culprit for our daily feeling of hunger.

The release of ghrelin is based on a circadian rhythm, which suggests that our bodies only crave food when they are used to receiving it.[50] We continue to eat because that's when we ate in the past.

---

50   Joseph LeSauter. "Stomach ghrelin-secreting cells as food-entrainable circadian clocks." *Proc Natl Acad Sci U S A*. Aug 11, 2009.

It might take a strong effort to avoid the hunger during the first two to four weeks, but afterward, it won't even register as being a problem. Most people consuming tea or coffee can blunt their appetite (usually in the morning) to fast for at least sixteen hours per day.[51]

During these first weeks and even thereafter, one of the common miscues is the feeling of hunger when our body actually needs water. Confusing dehydration with hunger is common and the effects on our brain immediate. For anyone adopting a fasting lifestyle, hydration and adequate water consumption are even more important than usual.

Water: Dehydration and the Brain

Try abstaining from food for a few days and it might be challenging, but it will hardly be fatal. Forego water for a few days, and it likely spells death.

Water is vital for the entire body, but the brain needs water (as it needs everything else) in a much higher quantity. Even the slightest dehydration can spell poor cognitive performance and long-term consequences.

Our brain is comprised of 75% water, which suggests we need a steady supply to maintain healthy cognitive function. The cells in our brain use water to produce energy and remove cellular waste.[52]

---

51 Recently, Dr. Rhonda Patrick has made the claim that anything altering metabolism (including tea and coffee) is considered breaking the fast. The jury is still out on this.

52 Public Library of Science. "Cells use water in nano-rotors to power energy conversion." *ScienceDaily*. August 4, 2010.

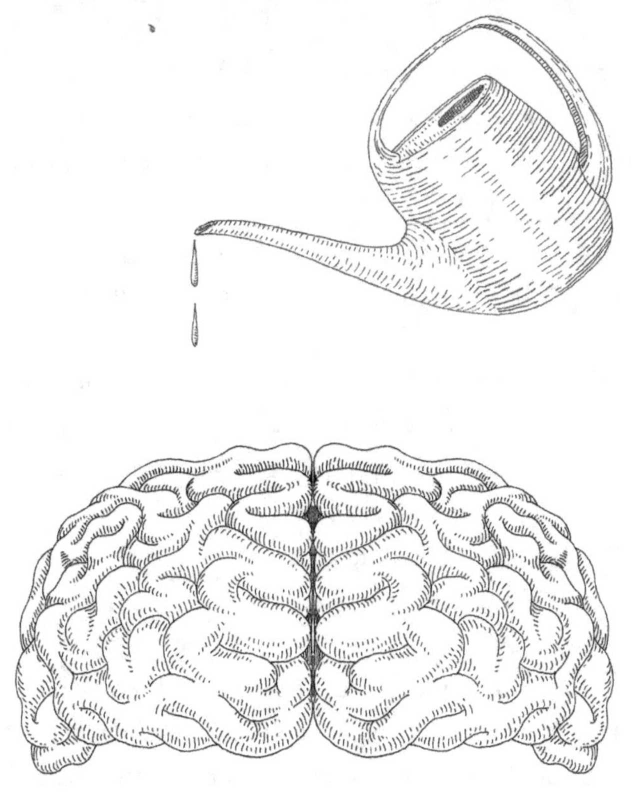

The exact role of water in our brain is still being researched, but advanced brain mapping techniques provide a basic understanding.

Data from fMRI scans showed that dehydration didn't necessarily affect cognitive performance, but it did increase the energy expenditure. Our brains have to work much harder (and thus burn out much quicker) when we are dehydrated.[53] Proper hydration prevents fatigue. Many nootropics enthusiasts seeking drugs to treat anti-fatigue and burnout can simply enhance mental stamina by hydrating properly.

---

53   Kempton MJ. "Dehydration affects brain structure and function in healthy adolescents." *Hum Brain Mapp*. Jan 2011.

According to other research, when we are dehydrated, cognitive function starts to decline. London researchers, led by Dr. Caroline Edwards, created a scenario in which participants engaged in mental tasks while dehydrated and then again when consuming adequate water. They found a 14% increase in cognitive performance and executive function when participants were adequately hydrated.[54]

Most strikingly, dehydration by as little as 2% can make a serious difference in mental capacity. This small deficit leads to poorer attention, reduced memory skills, and an inability to assess one's state.[55]

The difference of 2% hydration is no more than two to three ounces. That's only a few gulps of water!

If we do not properly hydrate ourselves, it doesn't matter what kind of nootropics or cognitive enhancers we consume. One of our first priorities must be to supply enough water to achieve our highest cognitive output.

Simplicity Diet

There are dozens of dietary trends and almost all have *some* merits. Each person is unique with specific neurochemical needs, but there are many commonalities from our shared ancestry.

A trending diet based on our ancestral needs, called Paleo or Primal, is what I primarily recommend and adhere to myself, though

---

54   Caroline J. Edmonds, "Subjective thirst moderates changes in speed of responding associated with water consumption". *Front. Hum. Neurosci.* July 16, 2013.

55   Adan A. "Cognitive performance and dehydration." *J Am Coll Nutr.* Apr 2012.

not strictly or dogmatically. Sometimes I eat rice; other times I indulge in brownies.

Based on our biological similarity with ancient ancestors, my suggested diet is one from ten- to twelve-thousand years ago (before the agricultural revolution), or at least two- to three-thousand years ago when we consumed whole grain agricultural products rather than highly refined and processed foods.

This diet usually includes lean protein (occasionally fatty cuts) and low to moderate fiber-filled carbohydrates, including plenty of vegetables of all sizes, colors, and shapes.

Most of our brain chemicals and neurotransmitters derive from the raw materials in our food. When we choose to eat amino acids (meat), it helps produce neurotransmitters. The essential vitamins and minerals in plants compliment the amino acids and provide the most sustainable cognitive enhancement that we can produce.

It seems that I have reiterated this point on every section throughout this "Beyond the Pill" piece, but *no nootropic can compensate for a poor diet*. If we consume powerful stimulant drugs while eating a poor diet, it opens us up to easier burnout or longer-term cognitive problems.

This needs to be neither complicated nor expensive. My lunch often resembles Dr. Dominic D'Agostino's (a proponent of a ketogenic diet and well-known researcher in scientific communities), who consumes canned sardines for a healthy source of protein and fat. I routinely crack open a can and eat the fish with a mixed green salad.

There are few dirty dishes, minimal costs, it's portable, and has a ton of nutrients.

This is more of a lifestyle than a diet. The difference is a lifelong, sustainable practice, which prioritizes cognitive performance in both the short and long-term. Sure, we can all go gluten and sugar-free for a time, but how sustainable is this? Instead, we should keep the 80 / 20 rule in mind and create lifelong habits.

Nutrient Shortcomings

Despite the simplicity of my dietary regimen, there are a few "greatest hits" I go back to on a regular basis. As our diets go (and that of most agricultural societies), we lack a few specific nutrients for optimal cognitive performance. Our focus on a few food sources (such as wheat and corn) has left us lacking in nutrition.

By contrast, our Comanche ancestors, who would routinely run buffalo off a cliff, relished a similar diet as most other hunter-gatherers: plenty of protein, some fats, and vegetables that they could find. The difference is, when Native Americans (or any hunter-gatherer people) ate meat, they consumed the whole animal.

If liver, brain, intestines, and kidneys sound unappealing, you're not alone. I've had my share of 'exotic' body parts, and most aren't exactly delectable. Unfortunately, as a result of our picky relationship with meat and its wide availability, we miss many nutrients our ancestors would have consumed. There are two deficiencies we should try to rectify:

1. Choline
2. Omega-3 (DHA / EPA)

The primary source of choline for our Comanche ancestors was organ meats. Now that we avoid these meats like the plague, choline can be a deficiency in some people. Eggs are a great way to remedy this problem.

For omega-3 fatty acids (DHA and EPA), the only effective source is fish. Algal DHA (the source of DHA for most fish) is great for vegans but lacks in EPA. The plant alternatives like flaxseed and walnuts contain alpha lipoic acid (ALA), which is an omega-3 the body converts into DHA. Unfortunately, the human body is unaccustomed to converting ALA to DHA, so we aren't efficient at doing so.

This is one of the reasons I suggest eating canned sardines. They offer plenty of protein but are also a cheap source of DHA and EPA. Salmon and other canned fish offer a more palatable option, but don't make the mistake of eating canned tuna more than once per week. It's a high-mercury fish, which could introduce more toxins than benefits.

Food Quality and Hype

If you have ever consumed a delicious, juicy, red strawberry, you've probably enjoyed the taste and the health benefits of fruit. Unfortunately, because of pesticides and genetic modifications, the benefits of some produce can be in question. If our favorite fruits and vegetables contain toxins because of modern agriculture, they will disrupt cognitive performance.

On the other hand, spending all our money on organic, free-range, all-natural, gluten-free granola can deplete our bank account rather quickly. Where are our efforts (and our cash) best applied?

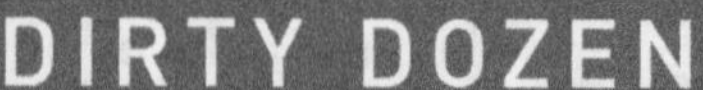

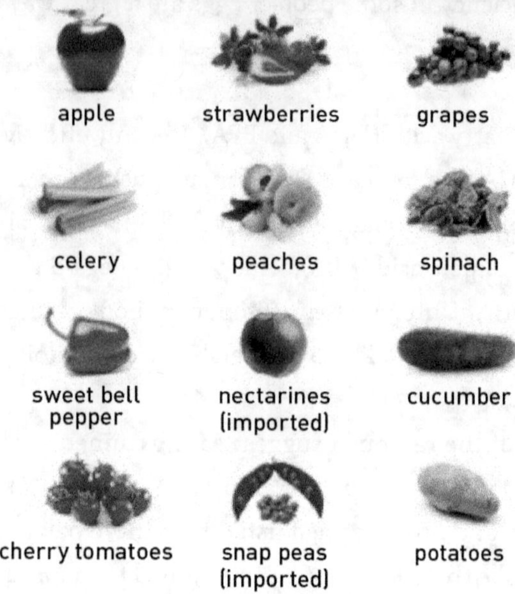

Sourcing meat-related products should be done with care, since the composition of the meat changes based on how the animal was raised. Grass-fed livestock or wild fish will yield far better health benefits, as they have balanced omega-3 and omega-6 fatty acid ratios.

A grass-fed animal will be leaner and provide our brains with more omega-3 fatty acids in the form of DHA and EPA, which have positive cognitive effects. When it comes to meat, don't skimp on the costs.

In the United States, pesticide residue on certain vegetables can be toxic for our health. While it will probably not lead to any

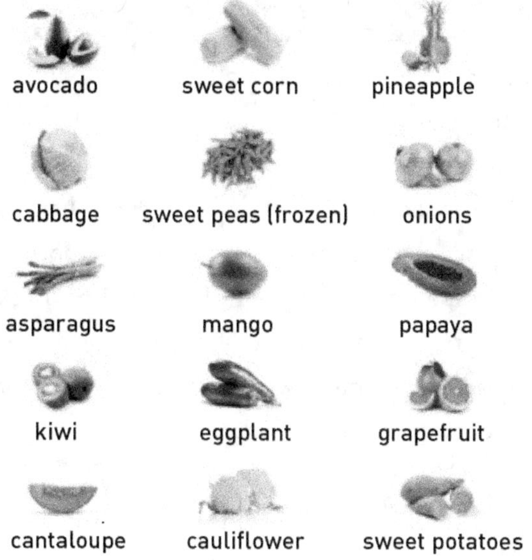

short-term side effects, the long-term implications of consuming these pesticides and chemicals are still unknown.

The "dirty dozen" list identifies the vegetables and fruits with the highest pesticide count due to the nature of their cultivation. As delicious as strawberries may be, they are unfortunately the worst on the dirty dozen list, with spinach not far behind.

While some concerns are valid, there is plenty of fear mongering and overhyped outrage. For example, blackberries grow naturally throughout Mexico. In fact, many landowners consider them like weeds so using pesticides is rarely necessary and neither are the organic blackberry products that we find in the grocery store.

Genetically modified foods aren't always bad either. Vegetables and fruits have been genetically modified for thousands of years. Modern GMO products are highly controversial and probably worthwhile to avoid, but a cautionary approach is more effective than a pessimistic one. To think all genetic modifications are bad is simply not true.

Our brain can only function at an elite level when its fuel is high quality and free from toxins. No amount of nootropics or smart drugs can compensate for a poor diet, despite what some people believe. Our first objective should be to outline a plan to consume healthier foods, drink more water, and eat responsibly—and only then seek nootropics further.

LIFESTYLE

Every day you live is essentially a string of habits. All of them impact our cognitive performance in some way. Even innocuous habits can have an important cause and effect on our brain.

When we shower, it can have an impact on our cognitive performance. A hot shower feels warm and stimulates brain chemicals like dopamine. A cold shower creates an adrenaline response with different effects.

Consider all the various habits we engage on a daily basis. We'd go insane trying to optimize every last one of them, but understanding the most important factors can help us to better incorporate meaningful habits into our day.

Move, Move, Move

Humans were meant to move. Following a more ancestral approach (of which I'm partial), humans did not sit around at desks all day. If you read no further, understand the importance of movement no matter the type. Whether it is walking or visiting the gym, frequent movement will alter our brain chemistry in ways that enhance performance and longevity.

General movement and exercise increase expression of BDNF, a neurochemical associated with memory formation and learning.[56] Exercise creates a cascade of responses, enhancing synaptic plasticity and even the size of some brain regions.[57] For the elderly, some form of exercise can be neuroprotective and reverse some

---

56   Fernando Gomez-Pinilla. "The Influence of Exercise on Cognitive Abilities." *Compr Physiol*. Jan 2013.

57   Ibid.

of the signs of aging via mechanisms like telomere length and autophagy.[58]

We're slowly beginning to understand the cognitive effects of exercise, but scientists see a broad range of chemical compounds upregulated during all manner of activity.

Consider the last time you exercised so vigorously it hurt. After periods of pain and exhaustion, there was probably a feeling of euphoria and positivity. When my girlfriend took me to a spin class, I struggled for ninety minutes on a bike. It felt terrible for my legs, but my mood was much higher after it was over. Thank you endorphins. These chemicals, often released with high intensity exercise, can improve mood, reduce pain,[59] and are associated with flow states.

Other brain chemicals like dopamine, noradrenaline, and serotonin are upregulated during almost all exercise,[60] which has short and long-term effects.

For the anxious, the neurochemistry associated with exercise can reduce symptoms of anxiety and enhance mood even for those who struggled with depression.[61]

---

58 He C. "Exercise-induced BCL2-regulated autophagy is required for muscle glucose homeostasis." *Nature*. Jan 18, 2012.

59 Adam S Sprouse-Blum. "Understanding Endorphins and Their Importance in Pain Management." *Hawaii Med J*. Mar 2010.

60 Tzu-Wei Lin. "Exercise Benefits Brain Function: The Monoamine Connection." *Brain Sci*. Mar 2013.

61 Mata J. "Acute exercise attenuates negative affect following repeated sad mood inductions in persons who have recovered from depression." *J Abnorm Psychol*. Feb 2013.

Like many of the lifestyle factors, exercise alters brain chemistry in a way that is sustainable for the long-term. Chemicals like dopamine and noradrenaline aren't uncommon, but taking nootropics to influence these can do so in an unnatural way. In contrast, exercise coaxes our brain to upregulate these neurochemicals itself rather than overriding our internal circuitry.

In general, we know some form of exercise will enhance cognitive performance, but it need not be a rigorous Crossfit workout. No matter our age or physical stature, there are exercise methodologies that are simple and effective for enhancing cognitive performance.

Walking is a fantastic example of a basic, non-challenging form of exercise almost everyone can do and experience benefits.

A Stanford study of one hundred and seventy-six participants found that walking could increase a person's creative output by around 60%.[62] These weren't long walks either; the study included five to fifteen-minute walking intervals and nothing more, which is something we can all implement into our lives.

Daniel Pardi, a cognitive neuroscience researcher at Stanford, developed an online platform called humanOS where users have an opportunity to track small, random bouts of exercise. His objective is to help people move more frequently throughout the day even in small intervals.

---

62 Marily Oppezzo, "Give Your Ideas Some Legs: The Positive Effect of Walking on Creative Thinking". *Journal of Experimental Psychology: Learning, Memory, and Cognition*. 2014.

For instance, it's easy to go for a twenty-minute walk when on a telephone call. Before hopping in the shower, do ten bodyweight squats. Try to include twenty push-ups before lunch.

According to Pardi, it all adds up, and spreading our movement more evenly throughout the week is not only easier for the busy professional but it also packs more of a long-term punch than a challenging workout.

This isn't a replacement for infrequent and heavy weightlifting sessions, but if you find that habit challenging to maintain, the small interval exercises can be useful. Nonetheless, a weight-training workout once or twice per week does have unique brain benefits.

The neurochemicals associated with heavy weight training can be great for cognitive enhancement. Cortisol, a brain chemical related to stress, can feel good and improve focus for some people, but it isn't necessarily something we want long-term. So don't over-do it.

A single heavy weight-training workout per week can be an effective regimen to enhance brain chemistry, stimulate the body's healthy stress response, and still avoid burnout. Doctor Doug McGuff has pioneered this training (or at least made it more popular) in his book *Body by Science*.[63]

The premise is to workout one time every seven to ten days, but do so with ultra-challenging heavy weights for a short duration. Offering the body an entire week of recovery ensures we'll become

------

63   Doug McGuff, Co-Author. *Body by Science*.

stronger every week without feeling overworked and burned out as other regimens often do.

Overworking the body doesn't happen only at the gym. If you have experienced the endorphins and increased mood from running long distances, it may be worthwhile to reconsider your techniques. While running can be healthy (especially if it truly makes you happy), it also takes a severe toll on the body. The brain gets a temporary cognitive boost, but over the long-term can cause fatigue.

The objective is to enhance our cognitive performance in the short-term while prolonging the longevity of our mental capacity longer into old age. A regimen of exercise is imperative to achieve this, but it need not be overly done.

Simply walking and exercising throughout the day in random intervals can be an effective supplement to one or two workouts per week.

Resting Our Eyes

Assuming the adage that humans are meant to sleep eight hours a day, we must dedicate a third of our lives to laying down horizontally for extended stretches at a time. Considering how little time we spend eating food and fulfilling other biological needs, this is a rather substantial investment of our time and energy.

A famous sleep researcher (if sleep researchers can be considered famous) once said: "If sleep doesn't serve some vital function, it is the biggest mistake evolution ever made." Yet even after decades, Allan Rechtschaffen and just about every other sleep researcher are unsure why exactly we sleep so long.

As of now, there are two prevailing theories, both of which can be true. While there are sub-theories and scientific inquiries under each of these two, they will sum up most of the sleep research until this point.

1. Memory consolidation and learning
2. Clearing the brain of the byproducts of thinking

Both of these are vital. The memory hypothesis has decades of research, but even the most-cited papers seem unsure of their findings.[64] Sleep processes engage newly formed neurons to solidify information and process memories.[65] There appears to be strong evidence of "sleep-dependent memory formation," which suggests much of our learning is formed during the restful hours of the night.

Two of the most important stages of development are the infant and adolescent periods, which both seem to require more sleep. While most readers are older, parents may be interested in learning that infants can sleep up to sixteen to eighteen hours per day to solidify their learning processes,[66] and that adolescents often experience reduced motivation and attention if sleep deprived.[67]

Consider a time when you have gone out with friends for a couple

---

64   Walker MP. "Sleep-dependent learning and memory consolidation." *Neuron*. Sep 30, 2004.

65   Maquet P. "The role of sleep in learning and memory." *Science*. Nov 2, 2001.

66   Amanda R. Tarullo. "Sleep and Infant Learning." *Infant Child Dev*. Jan 1, 2011.

67   Carskadon MA. "Sleep's effects on cognition and learning in adolescence." *Prog Brain Res*. 2011.

of drinks and socializing long into the night. Assuming you didn't consume too many martinis, the main reason you feel wrecked the next day is the lack of sleep and all the thinking you did during the day.

According to sleep researcher Dan Pardi, adenosine and TNF-alpha accumulate throughout a day of thinking (whether or not the brain engages in challenging work, it's always processing). These byproducts of thinking accumulate in the extracellular space between the neurons, which inhibit the speed of connections and make us feel sleepy.[68]

This is one of the reasons caffeine is so effective against sleep deprivation. When we consume caffeine, it acts as an adenosine receptor antagonist, which prevents adenosine from causing drowsiness.[69] Unfortunately, the caffeine only solves one small, short-term problem. Sleep is the only solution for a lack of sleep.

Maximizing the benefits of sleep for cognition isn't only a matter of sleeping longer. In fact, many people who require ten to twelve hours of sleep per night to feel comfortable are sleeping for longer periods to compensate for poor quality sleep.

There are three levers of sleep, which we can manipulate in order to wake up feeling refreshed, alert, and also protect our learning and memory formation.

68   Dan Pardi interview dated February 27, 2017.

69   Marla Rivera-Oliver. "Using caffeine and other adenosine receptor antagonists and agonists as therapeutic tools against neurodegenerative diseases: A review." *Life Sci.* Apr 17, 2014.

1. Timing
2. Duration
3. Intensity

One of the worst feelings is waking up during the middle of an intense and vivid dream. It is often (though not always) a sign of an interrupted REM (rapid eye movement) cycle, which is a type of deep sleep necessary for optimal mental performance. This example is a problem with timing, and may or may not be within our control.

Timing is a significant variable in our sleep quality because we generally sleep in approximately ninety-minute cycles and our circadian rhythm is finely tuned to our sleep schedule. If our alarm wakes us in the middle of a ninety-minute sleep cycle, there is, unfortunately, little that we can do.

Instead, if we set up our schedule to sleep for seven and a half or nine hours rather than eight, it might be more effective for these ninety-minute chunks. There is a high degree of variability so we each must find our own comfortable cycles.

The other aspect of timing is more within our control. Because humans are so dependent upon our circadian rhythm, a consistent bedtime and wake time can drastically improve sleep quality.

For example, if you usually go to bed at ten pm and wake at six am, then a night sleeping at two am and waking at ten am will not be as restorative. Even though the number of hours has remained the same in both examples, the circadian rhythm will prevent adequate sleep quality during the shifted sleep schedule.[70]

---

70   Dan Pardi, "Sleep and Circadian Rhythms." humanOS.me.

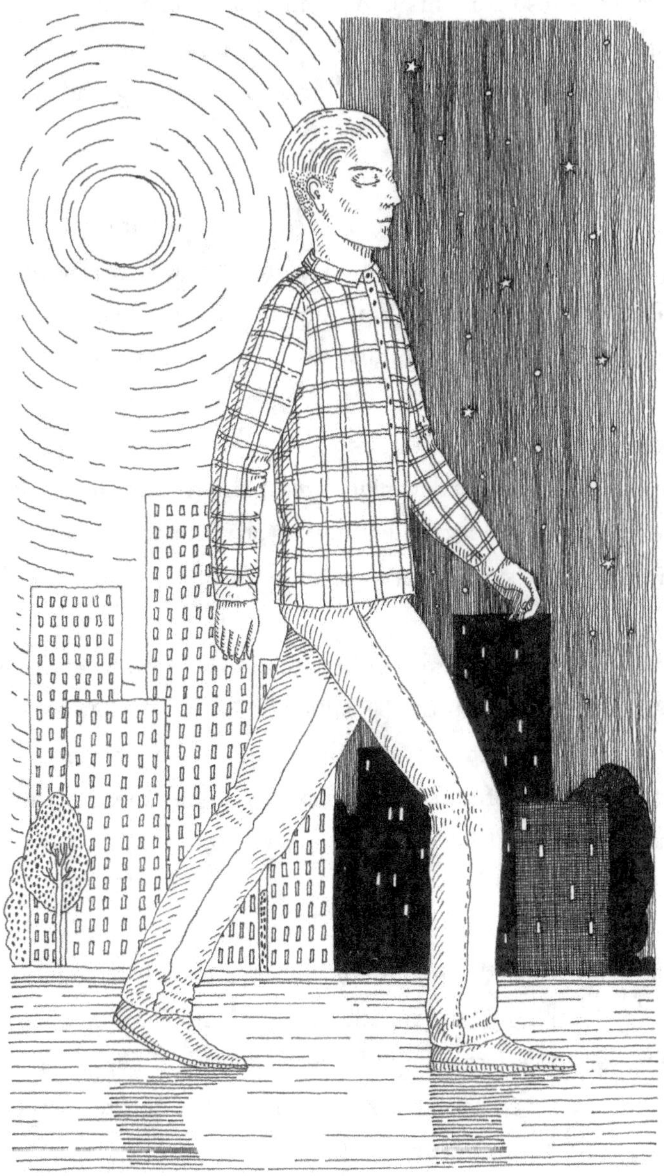

Of course, the result of this is not only poor sleep, but also poor wakefulness during the day, and poor health in general (long-term effects). The more regular we can keep our sleeping and waking schedule, the better.

The second lever for optimizing our sleep is the duration. This is the most obvious and basic method, which suggests we simply get more time in bed. The demands on our brain change from day to day, which means the duration we must sleep will fluctuate as well.

There are generalities for the number of hours we need to sleep on average, but a challenging day might prompt more sleep. It is a luxury to wake up on our own accord without an alarm and if this isn't possible, simply ensure sleep duration is long enough for the average day.

Time in bed isn't always the same as duration of sleep. Every morning I track my sleep with the S+ Personal Sleep Solution, which is a non-wearable device that tracks sleep via breathing patterns (recommended by a Stanford sleep researcher). Sometimes my time in bed is nine hours, but I only sleep for seven hours and forty-seven minutes.

Between sleep onset (the amount of time one requires to go to sleep) and random waking in the middle of the night, there is no telling how much sleep we actually get unless we track. I suggest the S+ from ResMed or even basic tracking devices like Fitbit to detect the time in bed and sleep duration.

The last lever to optimize our sleep quality is intensity, and it is amongst the hardest to manipulate. We cannot force ourselves into a deeper sleep, but we can maintain what Pardi considers adequate "sleep hygiene."

These include habits like receiving plenty of outdoor sunlight during the day (to provide signals to our circadian rhythm), reducing artificial light later at night, and maintaining adequately dark sleeping environments.

Light is the real key to enhanced sleep intensity. The more natural light we get during the day and less artificial light (especially blue light) we receive in the evening, the better our body can regulate our sleep.

For those who must use technology later into the evening, use programs and applications to block blue light, which mimics the light of the sky and disrupts the circadian rhythm. "Flux" works for Android and MacBook users and "Night Shift" is a useful setting on iPhones. Both block blue light on our devices, so we no longer have to wear ridiculously large, tinted sunglasses.

Every activity we engage in has an impact on our cognition. When we turn to nootropics instead of sleep, there is only so much we can do. If we avoid exercise and movement in favor of poor habits, it will harm our ability to concentrate, learn, and thrive. Ensuring basic lifestyle factors are in place will create an environment for cognitive enhancement long before a pill is needed.

Lifelong Learning

The human brain is constantly changing, but whether it is growing or decaying is largely up to us. Neurons and synaptic connections within the brain are pruned without use as we make room for new information and memories.

Humans learn in many ways, especially as we age. Even when we aren't trying to learn, our lifestyle habits inform our cognitive capacity. This section is both about engaging with activities that help us to learn and an accumulation of the other habits that impact cognitive performance, which has not yet been discussed.

Play is the Way

Marginalized to the eastern corner of Wyoming, the Comanche Native American tribe had little in the way of power. Before the mid-17th century, they were the black sheep of the plains Indians and altogether unimportant as a military or political power.

Within one hundred years, the Comanche went from their small corner of the American west to dominating tens of thousands of square miles, including the Dakotas in the North, Arkansas in the West, and Texas in the South. They vied for supremacy against some of the most well-known tribes, including the Navajo, Apache, and dozens of others.

In fact, by 1706, the Spanish settlements in present-day New Mexico created an alliance with the Apaches to ward off the Comanche threat, but without success.

The supremacy of the Comanche tribe throughout the plans of America was directly correlated to their culture of playing. Children at the age of four were given an old pack horse to ride. With no chores, Comanche boys were allowed the freedom to play with

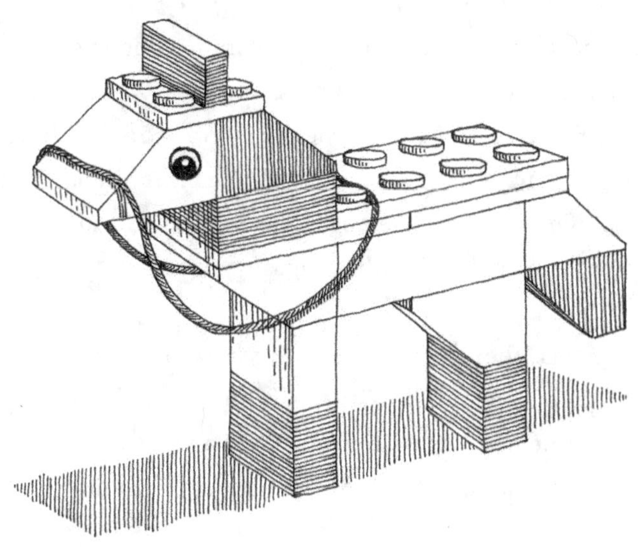

their friends and, more importantly, their horses. By six years of age, most boys were riding bareback, and by their early teens, they were expert horsemen.

From the evidence we have, the lives of Comanche boys revolved around playing with their horses. These mounted boys became men who could unleash twenty deadly arrows at a range of thirty yards before Spanish soldiers could fire and load one shot. Their military supremacy came from their horsemanship learned through play at an early age.

Much like the warrior Comanche, modern Silicon Valley is filled with coders and programmers who are self-taught tinkerers. Many of the most successful entrepreneurs who have started world-changing businesses learned to program by playing with code and building expertise as a result.

Play is the way that humans learn. Animal models suggest an "enriched environment" (e.g., toys, hamster wheel, and space) helps increase learning and memory formation by increasing neurogenesis in certain regions of the brain, such as the hippocampus.[71] Popular toys like Legos, Lincoln Logs, and others offer human children the same advantages.

Neurogenesis, the process of creating new brain cells, was once thought to be impossible after a certain age. Many of the animal models helped scientists realize it is a process that continues throughout life and particularly with the opportunity to play.[72][73]

Neurogenesis in the amygdala, a region of the brain housing our older and more fearful instincts, also helps to reduce symptoms of anxiety and depression.[74] Play can even negate the consequences of social isolation, a systemic problem of modern humans contributing to increased anxiety and depression rates.[75]

The Comanche knew little of these inner workings of the brain, and the tribe's success was, of course, more involved than simply children playing. Still, it's hard to dispute the connection between

---

71 Monteiro BM. "Enriched environment increases neurogenesis and improves social memory persistence in socially isolated adult mice." *Hippocampus*. Feb 2014.

72 Garthe A. "Mice in an enriched environment learn more flexibly because of adult hippocampal neurogenesis." *Hippocampus*. Feb 2016.

73 Speisman RB. "Environmental enrichment restores neurogenesis and rapid acquisition in aged rats." *Neurobiol Aging*. Jan 2013.

74 Okuda H. "Environmental enrichment stimulates progenitor cell proliferation in the amygdala." *J Neurosci Res*. Dec 2009.

75 Grippo AJ. "The effects of environmental enrichment on depressive and anxiety-relevant behaviors in socially isolated prairie voles." *Psychosom Med*. May 2014.

their rise to power and the role play provides for the learning process of children and adults.

A Mindful Approach

Yoga and meditation, both of which were thought of as "Eastern" pursuits for many decades, are becoming more mainstream. Nearly eighteen million Americans (or more) practice mindfulness daily,[76] and 44% of U.S. based businesses offer mindfulness training to cut healthcare costs and increase productivity.[77] Popular figures from Oprah to Hugh Jackman are making it more acceptable to take a mindful approach.

With more popularity comes more investment and businesses providing mindfulness services. Tim Ferriss, a famous biohacker and author of *The 4-Hour Body,* often refers to Headspace, an app created to guide meditation for the easily distracted.

Long since considered to be a mystical practice, modern brain scanning technologies are showing us what ascetics and monks have known for thousands of years. Mindfulness changes the brain in long-term ways.

Trekking through India, Dr. James Hardt has seen firsthand the changes that are possible through regular meditation. Focusing primarily on EEG machines, his Biocybernaut Institute recorded data from Zen meditators who have been practicing for forty years.

------

76   National Center for Health Statistics, 2015; "Uses of Complementary Health Approaches in the U.S.," National Center for Complementary and Integrative Health."

77   "Corporate Mindfulness Programs Grow in Popularity," National Business Group on Health and Fidelity, July 14, 2016.

These long-time practitioners had increased theta brain waves,[78] which are essential for learning and memory formation.

A lifetime of meditation may seem daunting, but it is surprisingly manageable. According to Harvard researcher, Dr. Sarah Lazar, only eight weeks of mindfulness practice for less than one hour per day is enough to increase markers of brain gray matter density.[79] Another study of hers suggested meditation was correlated with cortical thickness, which influenced emotional processing and feelings of empathy.[80]

This correlation translates into reduced anxiety, fewer symptoms of depression, and is usually the groundwork for an elevated mood. Beyond that, mindfulness can increase focus and concentration states during and after sessions.[81]

One thing both Hardt and Lazar have in common is brain imaging technology, which is helping a mainstream audience sift through esoteric, religious rituals, and understand the true benefits of the practice.

Luckily for us, the forty-year Zen meditators need not be our aspiration. Sitting quietly for hours on end during deep meditation isn't required when we cultivate a simple mindfulness practice.

---

78   Henrique Adam Pasquini. "Electrophysiological Correlates of Long-Term Soto Zen Meditation." *Biomed Res Int*. 2015.

79   Britta K. Hölzel. "Mindfulness practice leads to increases in regional brain gray matter density." *Psychiatry Res*. Jan 30, 2011.

80   Sara W. Lazar. "Meditation experience is associated with increased cortical thickness." *Neuroreport*. Nov 28, 2005.

81   Dunn BR. "Concentration and mindfulness meditations: unique forms of consciousness?" *Appl Psychophysiol Biofeedback*. Sep 1999.

Whereas meditation is usually done in a quiet environment and indoors with darkness, mindfulness can be practiced during an enjoyable walk, a yoga class, or even a few breaths while lying on the bed. Starting small gives us the confidence that we need to take on an ever-expanding practice.

Everything Matters

Our days are full of activities that impact our brain. From one habit to the next, we engage in behavior that alters our brain chemistry even if only temporarily. Obsessing about the cognitive impact of every move we make can drive us crazy—and it certainly is not my intention to suggest that you do so. The point is to understand that every action matters.

The amount of sunlight we receive on any given day or week affects our brain chemistry. Lacking in sunlight, we cannot take advantage of vitamin D, which is imperative for serotonin production and mood.[82] There are millions of people living in climates with little or no sun for months out of every year. This deficit may account for increased suicide risks in Scotland versus England where the former gets less sunlight during winter than the latter.[83]

Even our sexual habits can influence cognition. For men, pornography releases so much dopamine that it can lead to addiction.[84]

---

82   Patrick RP. "Vitamin D hormone regulates serotonin synthesis. Part 1: relevance for autism." *FASEB J.* Jun 2014.

83   Jong-Min Woo. "Seasonality of Suicidal Behavior." *Int J Environ Res Public Health.* Feb 2012.

84   Todd Love. "Neuroscience of Internet Pornography Addiction: A Review and Update." *Behav Sci.* Sep 2015.

An actual, non-pixelated, sexual interaction creates different chemicals, such as oxytocin and prolactin, which have differing cognitive effects.

When we are mindful that these habits can impact our mental performance, it allows us to course correct and modify as needed. Lifestyle patterns that fall out of line with our cognitive goals and aspirations can be removed from our lives only when we recognize them.

There is so much beyond the pill that needs our attention. It is true that we can pop a nootropic drug and see drastic increases in focus and concentration, but this is often short sighted. If we are using nootropics too often in the short-term, we do ourselves a disservice.

By approaching every aspect of life from our evolutionary psychology to relationships, diet, sleep and even disposition, we can perform optimally and also lead happier and more fulfilling lives.

NOOTROPICS

This is the stuff you have been waiting to see. You are now going to learn the fundamentals of using nootropics and smart drugs to improve your focus and concentration, sharpen your creativity, enhance your learning ability, and achieve more success in your life.

As powerful as nootropics can be, do not forget the previous lessons. As I've made it clear throughout, without the proper diet, exercise, and sleep habits, no nootropic will save the day.

Nootropics and smart drugs may be exciting, but they will always be secondary to the core concepts explained above. Let's get started.

Teach a Man to Fish

The obscure novel *Mrs. Dymond* was published in 1885, by an English woman named Anne Isabella Thackeray. She and her father, William Thackeray, were highly regarded writers during the Victorian era, though her work is scarcely known today outside of literary circles.

In the novel, she makes famous the phrase "give a man a fish, and you feed him for a day; show him how to catch fish, and you feed him for a lifetime."

That will be my approach here. While I could describe the scientific findings or create an encyclopedia of nootropic compounds, the research changes frequently. What we learn today will assuredly be different within a few years. The therapies explained will likely be surpassed by even greater inventions of which I'm not aware.

In order to make this book universally useful for years to come, the focus of this section will be to teach how nootropics should be evaluated. It will hopefully create a sense of self-reliance so that we may all find the tools that work best for us without falling victim to marketing hype or dangerous chemical substances.

What is a Nootropic?

Dr. Corneliu E. Giurgea coined the term "nootropic" in 1972, after discovering one of the more famous compounds called piracetam.[85] His strict definition suggests that nootropics should enhance learning and memory, protect the brain from toxins, and have few side effects.

Adderall, for example, would not be considered a nootropic. This stimulant-based drug dumps copious amounts of dopamine into the brain to create focus and attentiveness but has significant

---

85   Giurgea C. "Pharmacology of integrative activity of the brain. Attempt at nootropic concept in psychopharmacology." *Actual Pharmacol*. 1972.

side effects.[86] In fact, not only does Adderall (and similar amphet-amine-based drugs) have side effects, but they can also decrease mental performance in many un-prescribed users.[87]

As neuroscientist and founder of the Peak Brain Institute, Dr. Andrew Hill, told me in an interview, the two best use cases for nootropics are supporting healthy cognition and anti-aging long-term. According to Hill, "...the idea one would risk a drug or a compound with side effects to get a small boost in function is absurd."

This isn't common wisdom. Most people (sometimes even myself) will use nootropics interchangeably with compounds like smart drugs or cognitive enhancers (of which Adderall could be considered).

Knowing the distinction may seem like semantics, but it is not. The drugs have varying cognitive effects, and some are safer than others. It also points towards a more significant problem.

When we put our brains at risk from adverse side effects, it quickly becomes dangerous. Even worse is when people use smart drugs to achieve a "feeling" (such as euphoria), as is often the case with Adderall. It is akin to drug-seeking behavior even if disguised as self-improvement.

---

86   Shaheen E Lakhan. "Prescription stimulants in individuals with and without attention deficit hyperactivity disorder: misuse, cognitive impact, and adverse effects." *Brain Behav.* Sep 2012.

87   Wood S. "Psychostimulants and cognition: a continuum of behavioral and cognitive activation." *Pharmacol Rev.* Dec 16, 2013.

Instead, we must take a more skeptical approach to everything labeled a "nootropic" by marketing hype and anecdotal reports. The truth is, nootropics provide marginal benefits. If a placebo can provide around a 30% boost in our cognition (more on that below),[88] then nootropics and smart drugs have a high bar to hurdle.

Unfortunately, there aren't many peer-reviewed scientific studies on most nootropic compounds. As we'll discuss, there isn't enough money in nootropic research to make it worthwhile. To that end, we are on our own to wade through these waters carefully and with caution.

Nootropics Have No Morals

In 328 BC, near the unassuming present-day city of Samarkand, Uzbekistan, Alexander the Great sipped on a glass of wine. The banquet, celebrating his military accomplishments took a turn for the worst as alcohol continued to flow through the night.

Cleitus, a general in Alexander's army, had a deep personal connection with his king, forged when Alexander nearly died from a hammer blow from behind in the midst of hand-to-hand combat. If it were not for Cleitus, the Macedonian king would have been killed early in his campaigns. Quick thinking by Cleitus saved Alexander's life, and this created a strong bond between them.

Despite their long-standing friendship, that banquet in 328 BC turned into an argument between the men. As Alexander became

---

88   Price DD. "A comprehensive review of the placebo effect: recent advances and current thought." *Annu Rev Psychol*. 2008.

increasingly intoxicated, the argument escalated with both men shouting at one another. Alexander's rage and anger grew parallel to his drunkenness, and he plunged a dagger through Cleitus' heart.

Killing was nothing new to Alexander. For a man of his time, murder would have been easy to stomach. But not this one. Alexander grieved immensely.

Despite conquering much of the known world with the outnumbered Macedonian army, alcohol managed to get the best of the king. By age thirty-two, with more power than any other man on Earth, Alexander succumbed to an alcohol-related illness.[89] With his death, the empire he had built slowly started to decay. All as a result of his alcohol abuse.

Make no mistake; it was Alexander's fault. Some may blame alcohol, but chemical compounds have no morals.

There are millions of people worldwide who use alcohol as a way to relax or enjoy finer aspects of life. The same can be true of any substance or nootropic compound. A "good" nootropic can be used in a bad way just as a "bad" smart drug can have positive effects.

We must be aware of our internal dialogue and motivations. This is more important than the substance itself. Otherwise, nootropics

---

89   There is still debate about Alexander's death. Some evidence suggests he died of an alcohol-related illness and other data suggests it was typhoid fever. Sbarounis CN. "Did Alexander the Great die of acute pancreatitis". *J Clin Gastroenterol*. Jun 1997. and Cunha BA. "The death of Alexander the Great: malaria or typhoid fever?". *Infect Dis Clin North Am*. Mar 2004.

simply become recreational drugs that we use to escape reality just like alcohol or cocaine.

Does the voice in your head fearfully complain, "I'm behind on my work, and I'll never catch up to Joe without Adderall"? What about, "I have been really stressed lately, so I need some sleeping pills tonight"?

Both of these examples are internal dialogues that create an unhealthy, unsustainable, and even dangerous dynamic. "People seem to seek an effect, and this is very drug-seeking behavior," says Dr. Andrew Hill. "They're chasing some tiny incremental change…"

Are we looking at nootropics as a way to increase how we feel as though it were a recreational drug, or are we trying to create better brains for our future?

These are the types of questions we have to ask ourselves before becoming too engaged within the nootropic world. Plenty of Silicon Valley entrepreneurs, Wall Street executives, and avid biohackers find out the hard way that even a helpful compound can be abused.

This extends to both the synthetic drugs, of which we are warned to be skeptical, and the "all-natural" products so readily marketed to health-conscious individuals.

Natural isn't necessarily good. A product marketed as being "natural" doesn't say much about the efficacy or risks of the nootropic.

Vitamin D is an essential nutrient, of which up to 82% of the population is deficient.[90] As natural and vital as vitamin D supplements can be, anyone who consumes over 10,000 I.U. (only one to two times a normal dose) will die of toxicity.[91]

The same can be said for nootropics and drugs we consider to be "bad." Those without a need for it should avoid Adderall or other amphetamine-based drugs, but for those with severe impairment (akin to disability), the drug is life-changing and necessary.

Even a drug like nicotine, now vilified by the anti-smoking legislation popular in America and much of the west, isn't all bad. Brain fMRI imaging suggests nicotine can enhance short-term memory[92][93] and influence attentiveness.[94]

Drug compounds often considered "healthy" can be unhealthy and vice versa, but it depends highly upon our motivations. This kind of self-awareness before going into the world of nootropics can help us from making poor decisions.

------

90   Forrest KY. "Prevalence and correlates of vitamin D deficiency in US adults." *Nutr Res*. Jan 2011.

91   Parvaiz A. Koul. "Vitamin D Toxicity in Adults: A Case Series from an Area with Endemic Hypovitaminosis D." *Oman Med J*. May 2011.

92   Veena Kumari, "Cognitive effects of nicotine in humans: an fMRI study". *NeuroImage*. July 2003.

93   N. Sherwood. *Effects of Nicotine Gum on Short-Term Memory*. APS Advances in Pharmacological Sciences.

94   Levin ED. "Transdermal nicotine effects on attention." *Psychopharmacology*. Nov 1998.

Gaps in Science

The Scientific Revolution may have started in the 16th century, but there are plenty of gaps in our model of scientific research and the things we understand. The more scientific research we learn and verify, the more information there is to learn. Scientists open new rabbit holes, and we develop new hypotheses and theories.

The relatively new trend of cognitive enhancement is virtually unrepresented in the scientific literature. While we have plenty of scientific studies, our model of research is heavily geared toward curing disease, solving illness, and reducing pain. Almost thirty years ago, pharmaceutical company Elly Lilly began developing drugs to address Alzheimer's disease. The disease, which currently afflicts five million Americans and is estimated to increase to nearly fourteen million by 2050, is worth a lot of money to whoever fixes it. Nearly three billion dollars get spent annually on treating the symptoms of Alzheimer's rather than the underlying disease itself.[95]

Pain creates dollar signs for the large pharmaceutical companies. This is a great incentive for research. Neuroscientist Dr. Andrew Hill estimates a basic human trial costs five million dollars,[96] which is a huge investment for whoever is funding it. If the investment is for the collective knowledge of humanity, well, that's an altruistic and long-term return. If the investment is made with the intent to patent a drug and charge high markups for high profitability, it's going to appeal to a lot more people in the short term.

---

95   Robert Langreth and Cynthia Koons "After 190 Tries, Are We Any Closer to a Cure for Alzheimer's?" Bloomberg Businessweek, June 2016.

96   Interview with author conducted March, 2017.

With diseases like Alzheimer's wreaking havoc on individuals and disrupting the lives of entire families, it's no wonder most money gets funneled into fixing illness as opposed to helping mostly upper-middle-class entrepreneurs and professionals get a 5% to 10% boost in cognitive enhancement.

Even popular nootropic compounds, such as piracetam or noopept, have research predominantly focused on diseased patients. Of those human trials for piracetam, probably 10% to 20% or less focus on healthy adults in middle age, while the rest study elderly patients with and without cognitive impairment (dementia, Alzheimer's, etc.).

I, and others in the community, will cite this research on "sick" models many times because it helps us to understand the underlying mechanisms of a drug and demonstrate how it works. The problem is many of the obscure drugs and compounds (sometimes unapproved by the FDA) can measure their benefit in treating illness, but nobody knows whether they enhance our everyday baseline when we're already healthy.

Other shortcomings of relying too heavily on scientific literature are poor statistical analyses, special interest groups, cherry-picked data, and conflicts of interest.

In the early 2000s, the University of California at Berkeley supported research concluding that people eating "ready to eat cereal" were in better health than those who fasted or ate meat for breakfast. The irony of this finding was that Kellogg, one of the largest cereal manufacturers in the world, funded the study.[97] While the

---

97   Sungsoo Cho, Marion Dietrich. "The Effect of Breakfast Type on Total Daily Energy Intake and Body Mass Index: Results from the Third National Health and Nutrition Examination Survey." *J Am Coll Nutrition*, Aug 2003.

results may have been independent of any meddling, it's a conflict of interest that pervades the entire scientific community.

Other times the problem with scientific data is more overt. Statistical averages forget to include ranges, avoid medians, deviations, and all the other terms we dreaded in high school algebra. Most statistics can be manipulated for the purpose of anything and marketing for nootropics is no different.

Science Be Damned

My intention isn't to condemn science, but rather to shine a light on its misgivings. As marketing becomes more sophisticated, many businesses are turning to the use of manipulated science to sell us products (including nootropics).

Decades before the first nootropics, bodybuilders and strength enthusiasts were using performance-enhancing techniques for their bodies. Arnold Schwarzenegger, now one of the more famous bodybuilders of his era, was using supplements and dietary techniques untested by scientific literature. He, and athletes like him, found what worked best via their results and performance, science be damned.

In a podcast with Tim Ferriss, famed Olympic coach, Charles Poliquin, quipped that techniques he used thirty years ago are finally being validated by research today.[98] If he had waited until the science proved the results he was seeing, Poliquin pointed out, he would have been unable to train so many gold medal athletes.

------

98   The Tim Ferriss Show *"Charles Poliquin - His Favorite Mass-Building Program, His Nighttime Routine for Better Sleep, and Much More"* Dated November, 2016.

A similar ethos has pervaded many of the more courageous minds within the cognitive enhancement and nootropics space. Because there aren't many studies on healthy adults, and there are so many statistical problems and conflicts of interest with the evidence available, it's up to us to bridge the gap.

Empowered Responsibility

As we have seen, scientific literature can help, but it is not enough if we plan to tinker with our brain. Using nootropics and other techniques that alter brain chemistry is inherently riskier than doing nothing. More importantly, because our brain chemistry is unique, many drugs may prove ineffective despite plenty of health research and data.

To tease out which nootropics impact our brain, we must have data for ourselves. In 2007, *Wired* magazine ran a story dubbing the term "Quantified Self." In the article, technologists Kevin Kelly and Gary Wolf outline why individuals were interested in "self-knowledge through self-tracking."

Initially, a few eccentric Silicon Valley geeks tinkered with self-made devices and electronics, but over time the movement has grown considerably. In 2010, Gary Wolf spoke at TED about the Quantified Self movement, which boasts tens of thousands of participants who use dozens of devices.

These devices are making it easier for people to take empowered responsibility for their own physical and mental health. The process of quantifying our brain and cognitive performance is becoming not only cheaper and easier; it's becoming completely painless.

Devices are becoming more sophisticated, so they no longer need constant attention from the user. Instead, we can let it gather data without bothering us.

Writing this book, I visited the Peak Brain Institute in Los Angeles, California, where neuroscientist Dr. Andrew Hill provided me a basic understanding of how phenylpiracetam affects my cognition.

By using a QEEG (quantitative electroencephalograph), we were able to create a mind map of my brain on a day without any nootropics, and then again the second day while using phenylpiracetam.

In a procedure that only costs a couple hundred dollars, Dr. Hill was able to provide "…empirical evidence that phenylpiracetam increases focus, concentration, and quick-thinking…"

According to Hill, I was somewhat inattentive when I had no nootropic in my system (slight ADHD). When I had phenylpiracetam, my brain was more focused and sharpened by removing the inattention (rather than stimulants like caffeine or Adderall). Interestingly, the phenylpiracetam also boosted "fast alpha" brain waves, which are associated with flow states and creativity.

Not everyone has a few hundred dollars of disposable income to spend on mapping their brain while using nootropics, but the technology is becoming cheaper and more ubiquitous. A company called Muse has brought simple EEG models to market for only a couple hundred dollars. Now you can purchase one for yourself and gather data.

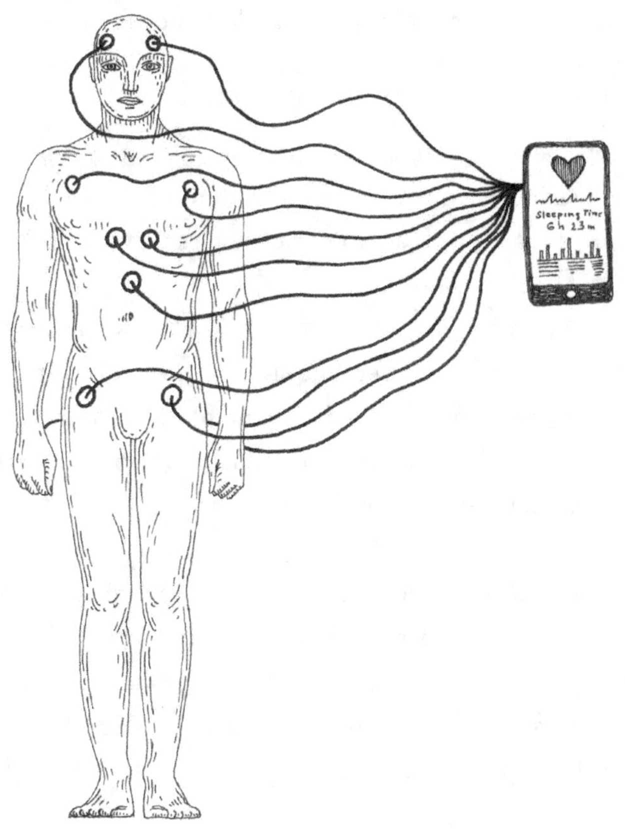

This is one of many exponentially growing technologies that will give us the power and responsibility to rule our destiny.

For centuries, consumers and laypeople have known less about our body and brain than a doctor, but that trend is changing. All of the doctors, therapists, and professionals are useful, but they are now advisors. We are each at the helm of our ship.

The data-driven crowd who enjoys capturing data and quantifying our biology will love the advancements that come over the next few years, but those with more modest means or interests can take responsibility as well.

Just consider the subjective experience of taking certain nootropics. Even analyzing ourselves through this personal lens is helpful to protect us and guide which nootropics we find most useful.

After taking a nootropic or substance, check in with yourself. Create a self-check system where you close your eyes, maintain a focus on your breath, and simply feel your body. Certain stimulants might keep us buzzing or over-stimulated, but it's only noticeable when we stop to check-in with ourselves.

For six months I experienced something that may be reminiscent of most high mental performers trying to achieve more with their time. In mid-2016, I was plagued with numerous attacks on my immune system. For six months I battled unshakeable congestion, warts on my feet that were rejecting every treatment, and I always felt sick.

Doctors couldn't help me with any of these symptoms. After getting CT scans and visiting my expensive naturopathic doctor for another perspective, everybody was still stumped.

At one point, things got so bad that my eyes were closing involuntarily during a 2:00 PM meeting with my friend. Sitting across the table from him, I remember fighting my closing eyelids over and over as he spoke.

After eliminating enough variables, I guessed my problems were caused by caffeine and the exhaustion that came with it. Even though I was only drinking a single cup per day, it was cold brew coffee, and I was extra sensitive.

After I had quit drinking coffee, all of the problems evaporated. My congestion cleared up, the warts lost the battle, and I felt better.

None of the doctors I saw, even with decades of experience and medical training, figured out that coffee was a potential culprit. It may have been something altogether different (as there is no empirical evidence that caffeine was the cause), but it taught me a valuable lesson nonetheless. Here was the moment I realized what could be achieved through empowered responsibility.

A commonly used compound like coffee can have a dramatic effect on our health and nootropics may have a greater impact. Being able to evaluate our own physical and mental state is imperative for our success. We must do the best we can with what is given to us. If that means merely checking-in to see how nootropics are affecting us, so be it.

What About Placebo?

Long considered the scourge of good science, a placebo is a story we tell ourselves (consciously or unconsciously) that affects how our brain and body function. A placebo is what makes food and wine taste better, higher education more effective, and even medical treatments work better.

In one study measuring cognitive performance and sleep, participants were asked to rate their sleep quality. The researchers then gave these participants a sleep score based on their self-reported sleep quality. Scientists gave some participants who received great sleep a poor sleep score while participants with poor sleep were given high sleep scores.[99]

Both groups were then handed cognitive tasks and, surprisingly, those given a placebo high sleep score from the scientists believed they had slept better and performed better on their cognitive tasks.

Another group of individuals in this study was merely told they had good sleep (even when they thought that they didn't) and it improved their cognitive performance. The scientists aptly concluded, "...mindset can influence cognitive states...suggesting a means of controlling one's health and cognition."

For whatever reason, modern discourse on nootropics and smart drugs positions the placebo effect in a negative light even though it is an incredibly powerful force in our favor. We have empirical evidence that when we feel as if something improves our mental performance, it does.

Many of the online communities are negative about the placebo effect and any potential benefits, but they are all missing a valuable tool for enhancing our cognitive performance.

It may seem like the advice I'm providing is akin to "just believe nootropics will help," which does not sound useful. My objective is not to tell anyone to "fake it," but only to point out that our

___

99   Draganich C. "Placebo sleep affects cognitive functioning." *J Exp Psychol Learn Mem Cogn*. May 2014.

common perspective about the placebo effect is lessening the efficacy of a powerful tool.

Radical Neurochemical Change: Psychedelics

In 2003, the British Broadcasting Company (BBC) produced a
show entitled *Peculiar Potions*, documenting some of nature's most
extreme concoctions. One clip showed a jaguar in South America
hallucinating with the yage plant, a vine that contains chemicals
like harmaline and other beta-carbolines.

Similar in experience to the native B caapi plant and their indige-
nous brew called ayahuasca, viewers wracked their brains to figure
out why animals were taking psychedelic drugs.

Author Ronald K Siegel explored many species that maintained
similar rituals, including dogs licking toads, goats eating psilocybin mushrooms, and baboons using an African brew called
iboga.[100]

From this research, Siegel has made some interesting conclusions
including one that suggests: "The pursuit of intoxication with
drugs is a primary motivational force in organisms."

Most of the animals that participate in this behavior are at risk for
side effects or accidents while tripping, but yet there is a biological
drive to alter their consciousness. Their objective is to shift their
perspective radically away from mundane habit patterns.

---

100 Ronald K Siegel, *Intoxication: The Universal Drive for Mind Altering Substances*, 1989.
     Pg. 11.

This process of "depatterning" helps animals that are repeating the same actions over and over to interrupt their behavior, but only strong psychedelic compounds can have the desired effect.[101]

These radical neurochemical changes in animals have the same advantages for humans. Traditional societies across the globe have used psychedelic substances to alter brain chemistry.

Native tribes in South America used ayahuasca; tribes in North America used mescaline, and even the ancient Greeks consumed *kykeon*, a dark black liquid many researchers believe was lysergic acid (a precursor to LSD).

Although hotly debated, Terence McKenna's "Stoned Ape Theory" even goes so far to suggest human evolution—and the brain, in particular—was tied to our ancestors finding and eating psilocybin mushrooms.

While this all sounds great in theory, most people are rightly unwilling to consume substances that are considered both illegal and intense experiences. Scientific research on psychedelic substances, such as LSD and psilocybin, had a nourishing few years during the 1960s and 70's, but was closed down for decades.

Within the past decade, we have seen a resurgence of scientific research, which has published encouraging findings about these psychedelic substances.

---

101 Giorgio Samorini, *Animals and Psychedelics: The Natural World and the Instinct to Alter Consciousness*, 2002. Pg 86.

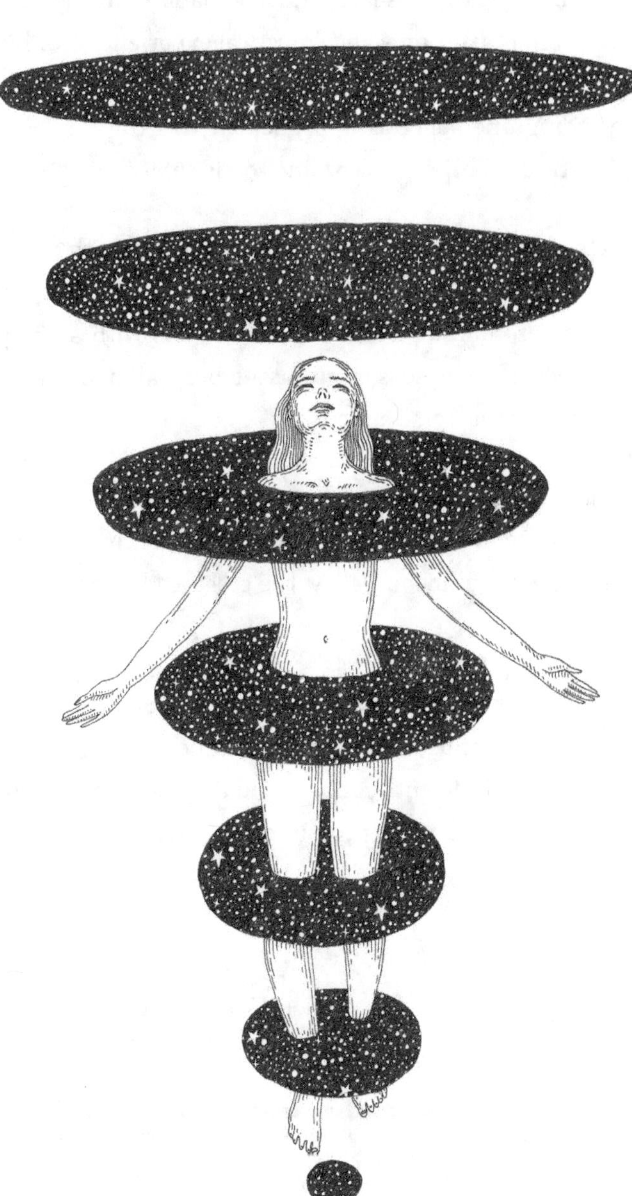

In 2006, Johns Hopkins researcher, Dr. Roland Griffiths began to study psilocybin mushrooms and "mystical experiences" of his participants.[102] Over the next decade, Griffiths published numerous works including one suggesting psilocybin was the catalyst for a top-five mystical experience according to his subjects.[103]

After fourteen months had passed, a single session with psilocybin increased their happiness and feelings of well-being. A Swiss doctor, Peter Gasser, administered LSD to patients with anxiety and depression, which reduced symptoms of both ailments with "no drug-related severe adverse effects."[104]

As the scientific community put more money and research into the topic, public perception started to change. But for creative technology entrepreneurs of Silicon Valley, the research has always lagged behind.

At Reed College, the unassuming and eccentric Steve Jobs walked barefoot around campus and maintained a peculiar diet. Working in a science lab intermittently, Jobs found Zen meditation and LSD. According to Jobs, "LSD was a profound experience, one of the most important things in my life."[105]

---

102 Griffiths RR. "Psilocybin can occasion mystical-type experiences having substantial and sustained personal meaning and spiritual significance." *Psychopharmacology*. Aug 2006.

103 Roland R. Griffiths. "Mystical-type experiences occasioned by psilocybin mediate the attribution of personal meaning and spiritual significance 14 months later." *J Psychopharmacol*. Aug 2008.

104 Peter Gasser, MD. "Safety and Efficacy of Lysergic Acid Diethylamide-Assisted Psychotherapy for Anxiety Associated With Life-threatening Diseases" *The Journal of Nervous and Mental Disease*. March 2014.

105 Walter Isaacson, *Steve Jobs*. 2011. Pg 41

The experiences with LSD were formative for Jobs, who later unveiled the iPhone and contributed greatly to modern technology. He recounted how LSD reinforced his belief that creating great things was far more important than making money, a hallmark of Jobs' thinking while at the helm of Apple and Pixar.

Steve Jobs was far from the only Silicon Valley executive using psychedelics during the "counterculture" era, and that same ethos pervades today.

According to author Tim Ferriss, the shift occurred "four or five years ago,"[106] as entrepreneurs and executives rekindled their love with psychedelics. He continued by suggesting that nearly all of the billionaires he knows in Silicon Valley are taking psychedelics to solve complex problems.

These renegade entrepreneurs aren't simply wishing on a prayer. In 1966, Dr. James Fadiman researched psychedelics for problem solving and creativity. In his experiment, twenty-seven male subjects in intellectual professions (including sixteen engineers, two mathematicians, two architects, and one engineer-physicist) brought a major work-related problem they hadn't solved over three months.

Administering a dose of mescaline, Dr. Fadiman discovered that 44.4% of his sample population (twelve out of twenty-seven people) had breakthrough solutions that became patents or other tangible assets.[107]

---

106 Steven Kotler and Jamie Wheal. *Stealing Fire*. 2017. Pg. 132 and 398.

107 Harman WW. "Psychedelic agents in creative problem-solving: a pilot study." *Psychol Rep*. Aug 1966.

The government shut down his and other psychedelic research shortly after, but the resurgence of modern studies soon validated some of these cognitive benefits. Although studied primarily for the purposes of relieving anxiety and depression, Dr. Carhart-Harris at Imperial College London has published findings using fMRI brain scans of patients while using psychedelic substances.

These brain scans, the first visual evidence of what psychedelics do in our brain, suggest psilocybin and LSD create freer communication pathways between regions of the brain that infrequently communicate.[108]

Harris found that areas of the brain associated with the sense of self and ego become so diminished that psychedelic experiences allow us to gain access to the unconscious mind. Within the right setting, these experiences provide radical neurological enhancement, which has long-standing and profound cognitive effects.

What Goes Up Must Come Down

The story goes that Sir Isaac Newton was sitting under an apple tree in his garden in 1666 when a fruit dropped on his head catalyzing a flash of insight. From this insight came the universal theory of gravity, which is one of the greatest scientific contributions of our time.

The story is undoubtedly embellished, but it emphasizes a phenomenon in physics that is universal: What goes up must come down. The same applies to our biology. When we tinker with

108 R.L. Carhart-Harris, M. Kaelen et al. "The paradoxical psychological effects of lysergic acid diethylamide (LSD)" *Cambridge University Press*. February, 2016.

our brain and change biochemistry, it's important to create sustainable cognitive enhancement as opposed to quick bursts and crashes.

Stimulant drugs are especially evident examples of this phenomenon when enhancing mental performance. Adderall, a drug commonly used to treat attention deficit disorder (ADHD), provides intense focus and concentration for many hours.[109]

When someone is correctly diagnosed with ADHD, this medication could be worth the risk of side effects. Impairment is a serious mental performance issue, and ADHD medication can help.

The problem is too many people are being medicated with these drugs, and even more are using Adderall off-label. Even Thomas Insel, the former National Institute of Mental Health director, believes children are being over-medicated.[110]

The downsides and risks of these amphetamine-based drugs are the perfect examples of the "what goes up must come down" concept.

Amphetamine-based drugs (like Adderall) create sleep disturbances even when one has stopped taking the substance.[111] What's

109 Dusan Kolar. "Treatment of adults with attention-deficit/hyperactivity disorder." *Neuropsychiatr Dis Treat*. Apr 2008.

110 Thomas Insel. *Post By Former NIMH Director Thomas Insel: Are Children Overmedicated?* June, 2014.

111 Gossop MR. "Amphetamine withdrawal and sleep disturbance." *Drug Alcohol Depend*. Oct-Nov 1982.

worse, many who take the drug experience debilitating withdrawal symptoms after they no longer use them. One scientific study concluded: "No medication is effective for treatment of amphetamine withdrawal."[112]

Even when a substance can help us to achieve better grades, stay focused in class, and perform mentally, we must always ask ourselves what the downside might be. As Tim Ferriss said when discussing the CILTEP nootropic stack, "there is no such thing as a biological free lunch."

The drugs comparatively safer than Adderall are still subject to this rule. Modafinil, a wakefulness agent and popular smart drug among Silicon Valley and Wall Street types, can be incredibly effective, but also has downsides. While some like to point out that the lower addiction potential and lack of euphoric feeling make it safer than amphetamine-based drugs,[113] it still modulates dopamine in an unsustainable way.[114]

Caffeine, a molecule beloved by the world over, can have drawbacks too. Consume too much and experience high blood pressure, heart rate, and crashes later in the day.[115] Many have experi-

---

112 Shoptaw SJ. "Treatment for amphetamine withdrawal." *Cochrane Database Syst Rev*. Apr 15, 2009.

113 Minzenberg MJ. "Modafinil: a review of neurochemical actions and effects on cognition." *Neuropsychopharmacology*. Jun 2008.

114 Nora D. Volkow, MD. "Effects of Modafinil on Dopamine and Dopamine Transporters in the Male Human Brain: Clinical Implications." *JAMA*. Mar 18, 2009.

115 Bloomer RJ. "Effects of 1,3-dimethylamylamine and caffeine alone or in combination on heart rate and blood pressure in healthy men and women." *Phys Sportsmed*. Sep 2011.

enced the jittery, anxious energy associated with caffeine, which is the other side of the focus and concentration coin.

An objective observer might find me unfairly targeting stimulants, but these drugs are where the concept is easiest to see. When we consume stimulants to get more from our brains, we must often face the unintended consequences later on.

The same can be true for even the most innocuous nootropic stacks. Many enthusiasts enjoy curcumin (a substance in turmeric root) to reduce inflammation and boost immune health. Combined with black pepper (piperine), these users try to maximize the absorption. Given that it has been commonly used in Ayurvedic medicine for thousands of years, many consider this a safe nootropic stack.

The unintended consequences may be harder to notice than stimulant-based drugs, but what goes up must come down. For piperine to increase the absorption of curcumin, it must reduce detoxifying enzymes. In the case of curcumin absorption, that's what we want. When it comes to other toxins and chemicals, it is not.

Jesse Lawler, the host of popular podcast *Smart Drug Smarts*, once shared a quote with me, which is compatible with my point: "Homeostatic equilibrium will not be denied."

Homeostasis is the balancing point within our brain and body, and having an equilibrium suggests we have a sense of balance. Our biology is always seeking homeostatic balance, which is why many nootropics seem to wear off over time. Our bodies and brains will adapt to many of the substances that we use—especially the ones that have noticeable "feelings" or affects.

Using these kinds of stimulants and drugs is not wrong, but it is a trade-off. There are many times where I'm willing to trade one day of ultra-fantastic deep work for a day of lethargy afterward. Without any judgment, these are all tools for us to achieve whatever goals we have set for ourselves. Of course, it wouldn't be prudent to warn readers without providing some type of solution.

When Sir Isaac Newton discovered the universal theory of gravity, he probably never imagined humans would break through this force and reach outer space. In the midst of World War II, German scientists finalized the V2 rocket, which was the first device capable of reaching space. In that instance, what went up didn't necessarily come down. Our technology gave us an exception to override the force of gravity.

Both humans and space rockets are complex systems, though humans are more complex. One of the best ways to avoid the biological trade-off with our brain chemistry is just to provide more of the raw materials we are missing so as to create neurochemicals ourselves versus an override of our existing circuitry.

When our western diets are an average ratio of 15:1 omega-6 to omega-3 fatty acids, suddenly consuming fish oil to balance the ratio and optimize our mental performance is a long-term endeavor with few adverse side effects. When we lack proper nutrition, such as vitamins and minerals, picking up the slack through supplementation comes with few drawbacks.

In addition to nootropics, which improve dietary and lifestyle deficiencies, there are ways to utilize smart drugs and even stimulants while mitigating some (though not all) of the drawbacks.

1. Take days off
2. Cycle nootropics
3. Vary mechanisms

Routine "off days" are useful for resetting our homeostatic equilibrium and preventing tolerance and withdrawal effects. During my off days, I still may take deficiency-based supplements, such as fish oil or coenzyme q10 (CoQ10), but no stimulants or focus enhancers.

Some people consider off days differently than I do and prefer to have no substance whatsoever. Whatever method works best to ensure that the brain and body have an opportunity to replenish neurotransmitters and other brain chemicals, do it.

Another useful approach is to cycle nootropic compounds regularly. Most people have experience drinking a cup of coffee, quickly graduating to needing two, and then feeling that coffee is a necessity of life rather than a means of optimizing it. Instead of falling victim to this common trend, use caffeine and similar stimulants no more than a few times per week, with a week or two off every quarter to reset tolerance entirely.

The final methodology requires understanding how nootropics improve our cognitive performance, but a few examples will suffice. Each drug or compound is a mechanism that creates the effect on our biology. When it comes to stimulation, caffeine blocks adenosine receptors and influences dopamine and adrenaline activity.

Phenylpiracetam (a member of the racetam family with a phenyl group), on the other hand, seems to increase focus and attention through the cholinergic system. When I visited the Peak Brain Institute, Dr. Hill showed empirical evidence that my brain reduces inattentiveness and increases focus and flow state activity in response to phenylpiracetam.

My brain may be unique in its response, but using this drug as a replacement for caffeine helps me to remain focused on work in a different way. Both drugs interact on varying systems of the brain and thus do not overly tax the same system.

When we focus our efforts primarily on rectifying deficiencies in our diet with nootropics, we can have a more sustainable hack for not only short-term brain function but also longevity and neuroprotection. Combined with the three tools mentioned above, we can increase our mental performance without overtaxing ourselves.

Safety

In early 2014, I met with a fellow nootropics enthusiast in Austin, Texas. Charles (not his real name) was trying many new compounds, and although it concerned me, he seemed a far superior chemist to me.

With his excitement written on his face, Charles described new chemical compounds he wanted to synthesize based on clinical trials. He showed me sublingual solutions of nootropics I had never heard of before. Eccentric for sure, but also intelligent.

It wasn't long after that he purchased a smart drug from a shady vendor. Its use resulted in seizures and a near-death visit to the emergency room. It was the first of many hospital visits.

As members of the nootropics community speculated on what might have caused the problem, lab results returned frightening results. The company had sent the wrong product. The egregious error was made worse by the difference in doses. He unknowingly consumed a dangerously high dose, which led to the emergency room visit.

A few months after that, Charles was dead. Whether the emergency visits and seizures were directly to blame for his death is unknown, but he was in his mid-thirties. The story always sits as a reminder of how dangerous nootropics and supplementation can be.

It isn't only a few bad apple smart drug companies that concern me. There are plenty of small, independent nootropic e-commerce stores with a reliable product and adequate safety precautions. There are also many popular retailers, who sell inferior quality products.

The attorney general of New York State accused Walgreens, Walmart, Target, and GNC of "selling fraudulent and potentially dangerous herbal supplements."[116] Reports found four out of five products did not contain any of the herbs listed on the bottles.

---

116 Anahad O'Connor. "New York Attorney General Targets Supplements at Major Retailers." *New York Times Blog*. February 3, 2015.

Replaced with cheap fillers and houseplants, many were potential allergy hazards or worse. If you assumed those four big-box retailers were trustworthy, think again.

There are three things you can do to protect yourself when buying nootropics and smart drugs:

1. Seek third party testing
2. Research community data
3. Use the "Shulgin method"

My first foray into the nootropics world was an online store. I saw that customers were scared about consuming nootropics with unknown provenance. Geoffrey Woo, the founder of Nootrobox, told me, "the chemical manufacturer in China doesn't really care, the middle man may be gray and loose with the safety concerns... and that scared me."[117]

When I founded my first nootropics store, the way around these fears was through independent third party testing. We sent our products to a laboratory; they completed an analysis, and provided heavy metals testing for less than three hundred dollars.

Once we had the results from our lab, we had peace of mind that we were selling products that were legitimate. We provided PDF results of the independent testing to pass that peace of mind to our customers.

------

117 Author interview with Geoffrey Woo dated March 7, 2017.

My company was successful quickly because of our transparency and safety precautions. The third party testing is still not the industry standard, but many of the best retailers provide this information for their users.

These days some reliable companies have internal third party testing with their own labs and machinery. While there is some conflict of interest, it is still safer than nothing.

The nootropics community is a great resource for collecting safety data on vendors. Reddit has around a hundred thousand members; Longecity has tens of thousands more. The experiences of others can inform purchase decisions.

If a vendor consistently provides poor quality products, they cannot be trusted. Another vendor may have consistently positive reviews, which suggests integrity. It is not foolproof, but it is an added layer of security.

Finally, there is the "Shulgin method" named after the American biochemist Alexander Shulgin. During his long career, he invented nearly two hundred and thirty psychedelic compounds. He is considered one of the most important figures in chemistry and psychopharmacology of the past few hundred years.

His "Shulgin method" allowed him to use the substances he tried for the first time safely. A microdose is the first step, which may yield no noticeable results, but can provide valuable allergy information.

After passing the microdose allergy test, you can then move up to a half-dose of the new substance to rule out a reaction to more of the substance. Finally, take a single dose of the recommended range.

By using nootropics incrementally, we can avoid drastic side effects such as the one Charles experienced. Even if a company sends the wrong product, we will reduce risk and quickly know whether it is safe by following the "Shulgin method."

Any consumable product has risks. Chipotle had E-Coli scares, and beef with mad cow disease killed dozens across Europe. Nootropics also have risks, but the steps I have outlined above can limit the downside and enhance our cognitive abilities with peace of mind.

Who's At Risk?

When a nootropics company sends the wrong product, everyone is at risk. However, there are a few circumstances when the risk is even greater even if we take the safety precautions mentioned above. Take extra care in these three specific situations:

1. Children under twenty-five years old
2. Taking more than one new nootropic
3. Experimental drugs

No matter your age, there are uncertainties involved with nootropics and smart drug supplementation. There are few long-term studies on the uses of these compounds. For children though, the effects are even riskier. Until the age of twenty-five, the human brain is still developing. A 2014 study in *Frontiers in Neuroscience* (a very reputable publication) concluded that many stimulants cause damage to brain development in early years.[118]

The authors cautioned against nootropic use (and specifically stimulants) as it risks damaging neurological growth and plasticity in the brain. Trading brain development and plasticity for more focus is not a good exchange for young people.

If you are under twenty-five, seriously consider halting nootropic usage (specifically stimulant-based drugs), and parents should keep this in mind with their developing children.

Another risk, no matter the age, is taking too many new nootropics at once. When we use the "Shulgin method" explained in the previous section, we can avoid dangerous situations, but only if we take a single nootropic compound. Some overly excited nootropics users purchase a dozen separate ingredients to build a "nootropic stack" without recognizing the interactions between the drugs.

These drug interactions can be dangerous. For example, more than one drug can interact and amplify the effects. It's best to try one at a time and in smaller doses. This may not always be possible (such as pre-made nootropic stacks), but at least use the "Shulgin method" if there are multiple ingredients so you can remain safe.

---

118 Kimberly R. Urban. "Performance enhancement at the cost of potential brain plasticity: neural ramifications of nootropic drugs in the healthy developing brain." *Front Syst Neurosci*. 2014.

Finally, most compounds considered nootropics are experimental in nature. Despite piracetam being discovered in the 1960s and studied in healthy adults, it is still experimental as it lacks as much research as other compounds or prescription drugs. However, there is a class of even more experimental drugs that can create added risk. Drugs like Semax have limited human evidence, and others like NSI 189 (an experimental antidepressant) or chromosome-altering drug Epitalon have little to no human evidence whatsoever. Most users are finding these drugs from a few vendors operating under the radar to serve a small market, but these products have far higher risks than others.

As the flip side of reward, the risks aren't necessarily a bad thing, but we want to limit the potential downside as much as possible. More importantly, we want to make sure we are taking conscious and well-informed risks if that is the route we decide to go. By adopting these precautions and understanding the landscape, we can make better cognitive enhancement decisions.

GETTING DOWN TO BUSINESS

Our scientific knowledge changes so frequently, it's better to learn the basics of these mind-altering compounds rather than make specific suggestions. There is a long human tradition of enhancing cognitive abilities through specific substances. Ayurvedic and traditional Chinese medicine have supplied eager merchants, artisans, and farmers with nootropic compounds for thousands of years.

These resources aren't difficult to find. Many alternative medicine anthologies are full of recommendations. Online forums and communities provide anecdotal information regarding doses and experiences of each compound.

Instead of regurgitating the available info ad nauseum, I'll approach the nitty-gritty of nootropics and cognitive enhancement by showing you the perspective most people don't want to talk about. The perspective where taking any and all smart drugs isn't always the best idea.

Focus vs. Creativity

As machines and artificial intelligence make repetitive jobs obsolete, creativity will become more important than ever. While hard work could formerly lead to prosperity and success, creativity is becoming the iron quality among business executives.

Out of fifteen hundred corporate leaders in sixty countries, over 60% said creativity was the most important leadership quality.[119] This came ahead of integrity, global thinking, or even dedication.

Hopping on the creativity bandwagon in 2013, the Red Bull Hacking Creativity project sought to study and better understand the skill. Scientists from the MIT Media Lab, TED Fellows, and numerous others, combined resources to analyze thirty-thousand research papers and interview hundreds of subject-matter experts.

According to Red Bull's Director of High Performance, Dr. Andy Walshe, it was "an impossible goal," but one bearing fruit in 2016.[120]

The crew found that creativity is essential for solving complex problems, such as poverty, energy shortages, and war.

With so much hope placed on creativity, it's no wonder many nootropics enthusiasts are trying to enhance this skill. Creativity is challenging to define, but working memory is an essential component.[121]

---

119 IBM 2010 Global CEO Study: Creativity Selected As Most Crucial Factor for Future Success.

120 Steven Kotler and Jamie Wheal. *Stealing Fire*. Pg 123 - 4

121 De Dreu CK. "Working memory benefits creative insight, musical improvisation, and original ideation through maintained task-focused attention." *Pers Soc Psychol Bull*. May 2012.

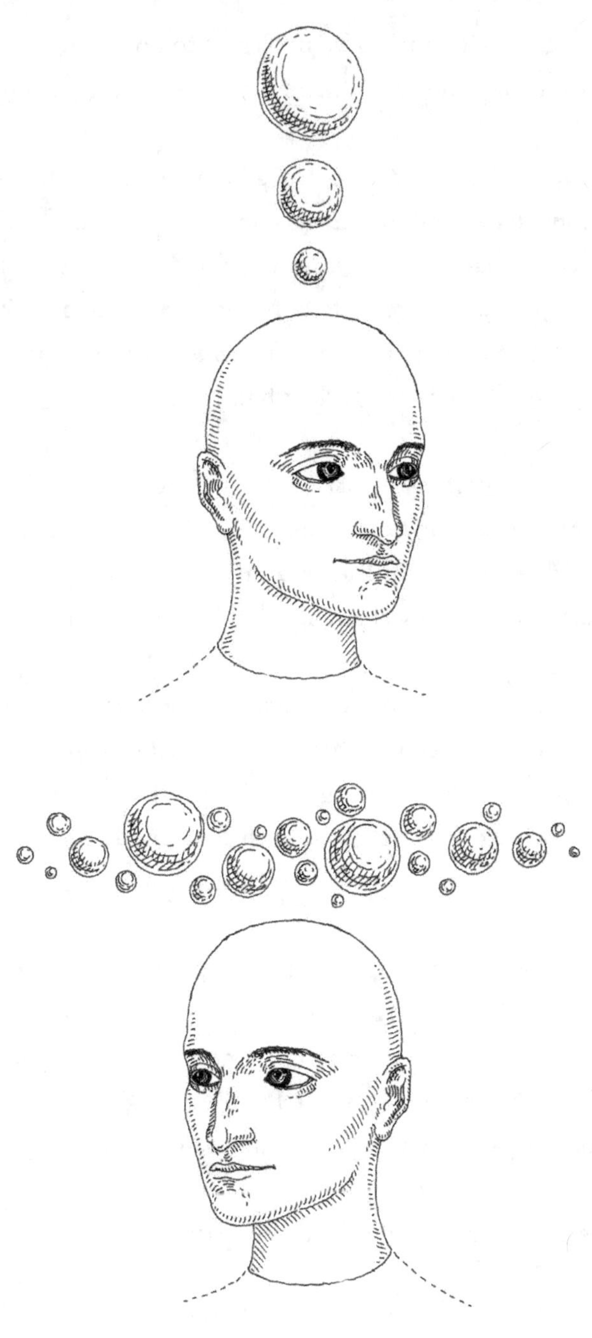

Increasing our working memory enables us to hold many ideas in our head at one time and combine them to form creative solutions.

Working memory is often referred synonymously with lateral thinking. Consider lateral thinking as horizontal thinking. It's the type of thinking that is spread out over a wide area. By contrast, focus and concentration are vertical thinking mechanisms. When we find a particular problem or task, we must focus on the singular problem and complete the task at hand.

If we consider creativity as horizontal and focus as vertical, it's easier to understand how different the two cognitive processes can be. That does not mean they are impossible to combine, but are often used for differing challenges.

There are few nootropics that can increase focus and concentration while at the same time enhancing creativity (working memory). One reason modafinil has grown in popularity is that it's a potent stimulant with benefits in both focus and creativity (by inducing adrenaline activity in the prefrontal cortex).[122]

Consuming different nootropics daily can prevent tolerance and withdrawals, and it will also allow customization for daily goals. A day filled with specific tasks (focus and concentration) may require a cup of coffee (caffeine) with some L-theanine. Aniracetam may be better for a separate day requiring creativity.

When bestselling author Derek Murphy writes fictional novels, he

---

122 Müller U. "Effects of modafinil on working memory processes in humans." *Psychopharmacology*. Dec 2004.

uses different nootropics for his varied needs. The only time he feels comfortable using modafinil is to create an outline for the story (requiring both creativity and concentration).

Flow states provide a pharmacological understanding of this combination of creativity and focus. According to flow researcher Steven Kotler, a short-term hack starts with a simple cup of coffee. This increases adrenaline and dopamine activity for focus and concentration, a twenty-minute walk can produce endorphins, and a joint (marijuana) can support lateral thinking through a chemical called anandamide.[123]

It's possible to combine creativity and focus, but not always easy or desirable to do so. Nootropic stacks should change daily and based upon the tasks of the day.

Stimulants

It's worth taking a moment to address the elephant in the room. Stimulants are the drugs of choice for most school children, overworked employees, and ambitious professionals. The problem with many stimulants, however, is that we don't fully recognize the effects of using the drugs.

Adderall (and Vyvanse, Ritalin, and numerous generic names) is an amphetamine-based drug. It is not the same as methamphetamine, but these drugs interact with the brain through similar mechanisms.

---

123 Joe Rogan Experience #873 - Steven Kotler. November 17, 2016.

The largest problem is that humans find it challenging to determine whether Adderall is improving cognitive performance or not. Most subjective experiences consider Adderall to improve cognitive function, but objective tests show this is not the case.[124] Not only do we have a weak understanding of our performance with these stimulants—many high performing individuals do worse.

A study of high cognitive performers found Adderall made their cognitive performance less than no drugs at all.[125] This is particularly interesting for the millions of off-label Adderall users in colleges and businesses worldwide.

There is another important concept involved with using stimulants called the Yerkes-Dodson Law. The relationship between being alert or highly focused and performance suggests there is a bell-curve response with stimulation. Too much stimulation (from either caffeine, Adderall or others) can cause poor performance due to high anxiety.

This graph will look different for each person, but it is an important measure to determine for oneself. Each person can gauge sensitivity with certain nootropics and smart drugs so as to optimize their results.

Stimulants, especially those that interact with dopaminergic or adrenergic systems in the brain, can be effective for alertness and

---

124 Ilieva I. "Objective and subjective cognitive enhancing effects of mixed amphetamine salts in healthy people." *Neuropharmacology*. Jan 2013.

125 Chou HH. "Amphetamine effects on MATRICS Consensus Cognitive Battery performance in healthy adults." *Psychopharmacology*. May 2013.

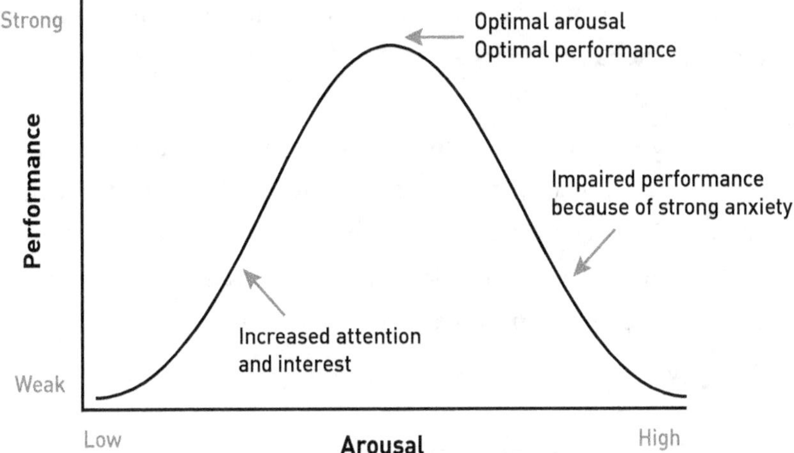

concentration, but come with a host of side effects. Unfortunately, nearly 11% of American children aged four to seventeen are prescribed some type of amphetamine-based drug and even more are using them off-label to keep up.[126] Armed with the knowledge about stimulants and their impact, hopefully, you can avoid making unsustainable decisions.

Preventing Decline

A shared endeavor amongst nootropics enthusiasts is preventing cognitive decline over time. This is a longer-term approach to cognitive enhancement than improving short-term creativity or concentration but is just as effective (if not more).

The life expectancy in America has jumped nearly ten years since 1960,[127] but many have a poor quality of life in their later years.

---

126 Centers for Disease Control and Prevention. "Attention-Deficit / Hyperactivity Disorder (ADHD): Data & Statistics" Accessed: July 18, 2017

127 The World Bank. Life expectancy at birth, total (years)

Memory ailments like senile dementia and Alzheimer's disease afflict millions worldwide.

Neuroprotection and preventing the symptoms of aging are ideal pursuits as human lifespan grows. This field is where much of the nootropic world started. Piracetam, a synthetic derivative of GABA (gamma-aminobutyric acid), was created in the 1960s and used successfully to improve aspects of cognition and memory in elderly people.[128]

Drugs from within this family, such as aniracetam and phenylpiracetam, have grown in popularity because of their creative and stimulating effects. Noopept is another powerful drug originally intended as a neuroprotective agent for sick, elderly patients.

As scientists studied the mechanisms of these nootropics, evidence suggested healthy adults could use them to great effect.

There is a low likelihood that these drugs will induce any stimulation or creativity. Because most beginners do not "feel" any mental or physical stimulation with neuroprotective compounds, they give up or quit taking nootropics altogether.

In studies on piracetam and bacopa monnieri, long-term dosing of the nootropics provides more positive results than a few uses.[129]

---

128 Waegemans T. "Clinical efficacy of piracetam in cognitive impairment: a meta-analysis." *Dement Geriatr Cogn Disord*. 2002.

129 Carlo Calabrese, N.D., M.P.H. "Effects of a Standardized Bacopa monnieri Extract on Cognitive Performance, Anxiety, and Depression in the Elderly: A Randomized, Double-Blind, Placebo-Controlled Trial." *J Altern Complement Med*. Jul 2008.

Users will need to cultivate a certain amount of trust in the drugs to sustain a longer practice with these neuroprotective agents.

Risk Averse Beginners

Some of the synthetic nootropic options mentioned above may be scary for beginners. Neuroprotection and enhancing cognitive performance in the most sustainable way possible comes mainly through the use of nutrients and related compounds.

Here are a few options for a beginner who may even fear the jittery, anxious energy that comes with caffeine:

1. CoQ10 and PQQ
2. Omega-3 DHA and EPA
3. Creatine monohydrate

These three options are long-term, sustainable, and mostly free from side effects or risks.

Coenzyme Q10 (CoQ10) and pyrroloquinoline quinone (PQQ) are compounds that improve mitochondrial health. CoQ10 is an enzyme common amongst most animals including humans. Most cells are filled with CoQ10, which produces more energy.[130] Over 95% of our energy comes through the process using CoQ10, which is why supplementing this coenzyme is a big win with few downsides.

Think back to high school biology class when you learned about

---

130 Ernster L. "Biochemical, physiological and medical aspects of ubiquinone function." *Biochim Biophys Acta*. May 24, 1995.

the mitochondria, also known as the "powerhouse" of the cell. Increasing our mitochondrial health may not feel like stimulating caffeine, but it targets the root of our problem rather than applying a Band-Aid.

By supporting the root of our energy production (within the cells), we gain a cascade of benefits. Healthier mitochondria translate to reduced inflammation,[131] can increase blood flow to the brain,[132] and are even attributed to a higher quality of life.[133]

The PQQ is another mitochondrial aid, but with a different mechanism. It's less understood than CoQ10 but generally thought to oxidize free radicals and toxins through a process called REDOX (reduction-oxidation reaction).[134] The downstream effects of PQQ changing these pathways are reduced markers of inflammation[135] and possible neuroprotective effects.[136]

---

131 Yubero-Serrano EM. "Mediterranean diet supplemented with coenzyme Q10 modifies the expression of proinflammatory and endoplasmic reticulum stress-related genes in elderly men and women." *J Gerontol A Biol Sci Med Sci*. Jan 2012.

132 Dai YL. "Reversal of mitochondrial dysfunction by coenzyme Q10 supplement improves endothelial function in patients with ischaemic left ventricular systolic dysfunction: a randomized controlled trial." *Atherosclerosis*. Jun 2011.

133 Lee YJ. "Effects of coenzyme Q10 on arterial stiffness, metabolic parameters, and fatigue in obese subjects: a double-blind randomized controlled study." *J Med Food*. Apr 2011.

134 Kamata H. "Redox regulation of cellular signalling." *Cell Signal*. Jan 1999.

135 Harris CB. "Dietary pyrroloquinoline quinone (PQQ) alters indicators of inflammation and mitochondrial-related metabolism in human subjects." *J Nutr Biochem*. Dec 2013.

136 Zhang Q. "Pyrroloquinoline quinine protects rat brain cortex against acute glutamate-induced neurotoxicity." *Neurochem Res*. Aug 2013.

Both CoQ10 and PQQ individually enhance mitochondrial support, but they are more effective together. A study of both compounds over twelve weeks showed increased memory and mental performance when used together, but not with either compound alone.[137]

Don't expect any sensations or stimulation from a stack of these two ingredients, but they theoretically will enhance cellular performance and improve cognition safely.

The second stack for risk-averse beginners is omega-3 fatty acids in the form of DHA and EPA (primarily fish oil). A high percentage of the human brain is comprised of DHA for historical reasons. Humans have mostly consumed freshwater fish and marine life for sustenance over hundreds of thousands of years.[138] Modern diets lack in fish, and most people are deficient in a nutrient, which is imperative for adequate brain function.

Again, the reasoning behind DHA and EPA supplementation begins at the cellular level. When the ratio of omega-3 and omega-6 fatty acids is balanced in the cell, it interacts appropriately with hormones. If the ratio is skewed towards omega-6 fatty acids (average western diets are 15-20:1 omega-6 to omega-3), the cell walls will be short, brittle and less flexible. The result is poor cellular function.[139]

---

137 Kei Ohwada. "Pyrroloquinoline Quinone (PQQ) Prevents Cognitive Deficit Caused by Oxidative Stress in Rats." *J Clin Biochem Nutr*. Jan 2008.

138 Joanne Bradbury. "Docosahexaenoic Acid (DHA): An Ancient Nutrient for the Modern Human Brain." *Nutrients*. May 2011.

139 Doug McGuff and John Little. *Body by Science*. Page 192

Optimizing the function of the cell (as with CoQ10 and PQQ) creates a cascade of benefits. Fish oil (the primary source of DHA / EPA) can reduce inflammation and protect neurons.[140] Other studies show anti-anxiety benefits[141] and even improved memory formation and learning.[142]

If you cannot eat more fish, supplemental fish oil will help achieve the optimal one-to-one ratio of omega-3 fatty acids. Even vegans can consume algal DHA, which is the source of DHA for all fish as well.

The final selection for risk-averse beginners is creatine monohydrate. All mammals have creatine, which is a molecule that aids in mitochondrial health. Creatine helps increase ATP (energy) within the cells, but it does not discriminate body or brain. For the same reason creatine is an effective strength building tool for bodybuilders and athletes, it can also help the brain.[143]

The downstream effects of added energy through creatine are greater for vegans and vegetarians, who consume no creatine via

---

140 Luchtman DW. "Cognitive enhancement by omega-3 fatty acids from child-hood to old age: findings from animal and clinical studies." *Neuropharmacology*. Jan 2013.

141 Kiecolt-Glaser JK. "Omega-3 supplementation lowers inflammation and anxiety in medical students: a randomized controlled trial." *Brain Behav Immun*. Nov 2011.

142 Kidd PM. "Omega-3 DHA and EPA for cognition, behavior, and mood: clinical findings and structural-functional synergies with cell membrane phospholipids." *Altern Med Rev*. Sep 2007.

143 Lawler JM. "Direct antioxidant properties of creatine." *Biochem Biophys Res Commun*. Jan 11, 2002.

meat products.[144] The effects on young adults and elderly are helpful for neuroprotection, increasing aspects of cognition (such as memory), and preventing neurological decline (such as Alzheimer's disease).[145]

A common myth suggests creatine is unhealthy for the kidneys, but this is only true for users with existing impairment. Even in those cases, there is conflicting evidence suggesting no adverse side effects for the kidneys (even while they are under stress).[146] For healthy adults, the risks are low while the benefits are high.

None of these options will drastically increase daily output, creativity, or concentration, but will aid in small, incremental cognitive enhancement. By using these (and many other) compounds that improve the cells in our body and brain, we create a cascade of benefits that support our short and long-term goals.

144　Rawson ES. "Creatine supplementation does not improve cognitive function in young adults." *Physiol Behav*. Sep 3, 2008.

145　Wallimann T. "The creatine kinase system and pleiotropic effects of creatine." *Amino Acids*. May 2011.

146　Shefner JM. "A clinical trial of creatine in ALS." *Neurology*. Nov 9, 2004.

PIECING IT ALL TOGETHER

We all want a quick fix. Humans desire shortcuts. Bill Gates, the paragon of entrepreneurs and business leaders, once said: "I will always choose a lazy person to do a difficult job... because he will find an easy way to do it."

As humans, the desire to take shortcuts became hardwired into our brain over hundreds of thousands of years, and our tool-making ability has made it possible to work smarter instead of harder. We aren't "wrong" or "bad" for seeking hacks, boosts, or timesavers; we are following human nature.

Sometimes these shortcuts don't go as planned. When hunter-gatherers stopped roaming the plains and instead started farming, our ancestors thought they had taken a shortcut. As author Yuval Noah Harari points out, this made humanity more militant, warlike, and less happy than before.[147]

------

147 Yuval Noah Harari. *Sapiens: A Brief History of Mankind.*

The same is true of our brains. We may seek a shortcut that seems to work in the short-term, but it does not necessarily translate into a long-term plan to achieve our best.

The image of Wall Street executives and Silicon Valley entrepreneurs working themselves to the bone and consuming smart drugs to get ahead has been imprinted on the mainstream consciousness. The current "movers and shakers" seem to be energized, productive, and successful, but many are over-medicating with smart drugs in an unsustainable way.

Tim Ferriss has experimented with many nootropics including some of the most potent drugs on (and off) the marketplace. In the past year, his temperament towards nootropics has changed considerably. He has moved away from highly stimulating, short-term smart drugs and more towards long-term, sustainable supplementation. He's reached the same conclusion I have: *slow and steady wins the race.*

A metaphor for these two contrasting styles of smart drug usage is the tale of the tortoise and the hare. Nearly every child has heard this story. The fable speaks to a common human experience, which has stood the test of time.

Will the brazen, boastful, and fast-paced hare win or the slow and steady tortoise? As children know, the hare takes a nap near the finish line, and the tortoise slowly crosses the finish line for the win.

The parallels within the smart drug world are no different. Fast-paced executives hurry to and from meetings for days, months, or sometimes years, fueled by caffeine and other stimulants. Burn-out and depression are so common among entrepreneurs, especially at the highest level, that the slow and steady path is often more effective.

The approach of the tortoise is more constant, longer-term, and sustainable. That doesn't mean we cannot use the hare approach now and again, but it ought to be within the framework of slow and steady. The new approach I advocate for nootropics and smart drug usage is 30% hare and 70% tortoise.

The largest efforts are made towards healthy lifestyle habits, such as diet, sleep, and community. We take days off from nootropics, vary the mechanisms, and cycle various smart drugs to avoid tolerance and withdrawal effects.

We still utilize powerful smart drugs for enhancing our concentration and achieving our fullest potential, but we do so consciously and with care. Even highly powered psychedelics, such as LSD or psilocybin, can play a major role within our regimen when used correctly.

Tools to improve our cognitive enhancement do not affect only us. When we emphasize the right nootropics and a lifestyle geared towards optimizing our brain, we become happier, more enjoyable people for our co-workers, friends, and family. We can achieve more over our lifetime and impact the world around us in a more positive way.

The World is Waiting

As of March 2016, the Google driverless automobile team recorded that their fleet of vehicles traveled 1,500,000 miles with only a handful of accidents.[148] Far safer than error-prone humans, artificial intelligence was being used to radically change human transportation. Beyond driverless cars, Google is working on virtual reality platforms, advanced robotics, and just about any futuristic technology you can think of.

Not far away from Google headquarters, Elon Musk is developing transportation technologies of science fiction lore. The Tesla electric cars are more advanced than any others and Musk is actively campaigning to settle Mars with a human colony through his private space company.

What Elon Musk and Google co-founder Sergey Brin both have in common is their emphasis on optimizing mental performance. Both men, along with thousands of Silicon Valley executives, attend the mind-altering infused event called Burning Man every year.[149] In and outside of this annual festival, the best and brightest are finding every way possible to enhance their cognitive abilities and set up humans for a more advanced future.

To drop into a flow state, Brin enjoys a "looping swing" built by Flow Genome Project founders Steven Kotler and Jamie Wheal. Musk is exploring how to enhance the brain through a computer interface (imagine half-brain, half-computer) in a company called Neuralink. Both paragons of innovation and success see the vast potential of brain optimization.

---

148 Google Self-Driving Car Project Monthly Report (March 2016).

149 Steven Kotler and Jamie Wheal. *Stealing Fire*.

You can be part of these innovations. Many of the tools Sergey Brin, Elon Musk, and other high performance individuals have at their disposal are becoming widely available to the public.

When present-day U.S. military snipers use tDCS to increase learning ability by 230%, they use the same tools we can make ourselves for less than $50. With services like 23andme, we can access our own genetic code for less than $200 and simple QEEG brain maps require less time and money than a doctor's visit only a decade ago.

Whether your desire is to make a contribution to science, art, business, or charitable organizations, we can better accomplish these world changing goals through cognitive enhancement. A healthy foundation of adequate sleep, diet, exercise, and mindset gives us a strong place to start experimenting with nootropics and other brain enhancing technologies.

With the essentials provided in this book, you can take the next steps towards mastering cognitive abilities. Simply visit *www. aheadabovebook.com/resources* to find more in-depth action steps and strategies.

Small changes to the human brain make big differences in our abilities as a species. As we saw in the 17th and 18th centuries, the introduction of coffee helped create some of the greatest scientific and philosophical contributions to humanity. With the democratization of new technologies, we will witness mankind's flourishing once again.

www.ingramcontent.com/pod-product-compliance
Lightning Source LLC
Chambersburg PA
CBHW071218240726
48654CB00009B/838